John Brookfield

MASTERY

OF

HAND

STRENGTH

FOREWORD BY RANDALL J. STROSSEN, PH.D.

———

IronMind® Enterprises, Inc.
Nevada City, California

Mastery of Hand Strength
© 1995 IronMind Enterprises, Inc.

Cataloging in Publication Data
Brookfield, John—
Mastery of hand strength
1. Fitness training for sports   2. Weight lifting
1995   613.711 95-078894
ISBN 0-926888-03-X

Book and cover design by Tony Agpoon, Sausalito, California

Published in the United States of America
IronMind Enterprises, Inc., P.O. Box 1228, Nevada City, CA 95959

Printed in the U.S.A. First Edition
20 19 18 17 16 15

To my wife Sherry, for her encouragement and understanding.

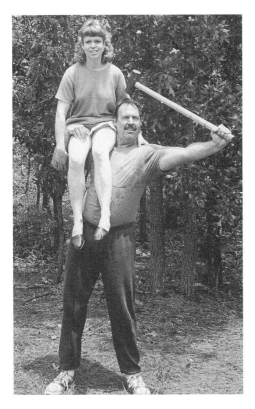

John Brookfield toys with a 10-lb. sledgehammer lever lift, with Sherry on his shoulder. Photo by Erica McArthur.

Other IronMind Enterprises, Inc. publications:

SUPER SQUATS: How to Gain 30 Pounds of Muscle in 6 Weeks
 by Randall J. Strossen, Ph.D.

The Complete Keys to Progress by John McCallum, edited by Randall J. Strossen, Ph.D.

IronMind: Stronger Minds, Stronger Bodies by Randall J. Strossen, Ph.D.

MILO: A Journal for Serious Strength Athletes, Randall J. Strossen, Ph.D., Publisher and
 Editor-in-chief

Powerlifting Basics, Texas-style: The Adventures of Lope Delk by Paul Kelso

Of Stones and Strength by Steve Jeck and Peter Martin

Sons of Samson, Volume 2 Profiles by David Webster

Rock Iron Steel: The Book of Strength by Steve Justa

Paul Anderson: The Mightiest Minister by Randall J. Strossen, Ph.D.

Louis Cyr: Amazing Canadian by Ben Weider, CM

Training with Cables for Strength by John Brookfield

The Grip Master's Manual by John Brookfield

Captains of Crush® Grippers: What They Are and How to Close Them
 by Randall J. Strossen, Ph.D., J. B. Kinney and Nathan Holle

Winning Ways: How to Succeed In the Gym and Out by Randall J. Strossen, Ph.D.

The Complete Sandbag Training Course by Brian Jones

Bodyweight Exercises for Extraordinary Strength by Brad Johnson

To order additional copies of *Mastery of Hand Strength* or for a catalog of IronMind
Enterprises, Inc. publications and products, please contact:

> IronMind Enterprises, Inc.
> P. O. Box 1228
> Nevada City, CA 95959 USA
> tel: (530) 265-6725
> fax: (530) 265-4876
> website: www.ironmind.com
> e-mail: sales@ironmind.com

Contents

One of the real pleasures of working at IronMind® Enterprises, Inc. is that you can rub elbows with the strongest people around, and when they also turn out to be nice guys, it doesn't get much better.

John Brookfield first called us up about six years ago, introducing himself as a professional strongman. John was calling because Richard Sorin had told him about our handgrippers, and since John, several years before that, had set himself the goal of developing the strongest hands in the world, you can imagine his reaction to our #3 gripper.

Over the years since then, I have spent countless hours talking with John and have followed his career as he progressed from someone who was stymied by our #3 to the second person to close it. Not content with having become a certified member of the "Captains of Crush™," this was only the beginning for John.

Since then, a handful of men in the world have closed our #3 gripper, and of those that we know of who have tried our #4 gripper, none gets the handles beyond about parallel. As we go to press, John Brookfield, while steadying the gripper with a finger from his free hand, has fully closed the #4!!! This gripper is so tough that most really strong men will barely budge it.

But that's only the beginning. John has not only become the only man in the world besides Richard Sorin to lift Richard's "blob" (half a York 100-pound cast dumbbell) with a pinch grip, but he has also done something nobody else ever has—he has lifted it with an additional five pounds hanging from it. And if you're interested in bending nails, tearing cards, etc., we'll just make it simple and say that for the last several years, we've never heard of anyone remotely comparable to John, and the really scary part is that John just keeps getting better and better.

We could go on and on about what John can do with his hands, but the real point is that John got that way because he is immensely dedicated to his craft and his imagination, as far as training goes, is boundless. I can guarantee you that I have never met anyone with John's enthusiasm and creativity when it comes to hand training.

So when we say you now have a chance to learn from a master of hand strength—John Brookfield—we're not blowing smoke. In fact, if you want to learn how to get stronger hands, look no further, because this is the best book ever written on the subject. Period.

This book will introduce you to some of the leading gripmasters, past and present, and even tell you how to make most of the equipment you will need to develop a world-class grip, but its real strength is its wealth of training information. I am firmly convinced that the reason why John has reached the pinnacle of the hand strength world is because he is so enthusiastic about training and is forever coming up with new exercises.

You cannot read this book with becoming infected with John's zest for hand strength and you will undoubtedly meet many, many hand-strength exercises you never even heard of before. The result? If you follow John's advice, you are virtually certain of taking your own hand strength to new heights.

Randall J. Strossen, Ph.D.
President
IronMind® Enterprises, Inc.
Nevada City, California

John Brookfield

MASTERY

OF

HAND

STRENGTH

Have you ever wondered how you could develop a powerful grip—not just a good grip, but a world class grip that could be used for almost any endeavor? A grip that could be used to bend nails, hit the farthest baseball, chop wood without your hands getting tired, or simply just give a firm, powerful handshake. I think most people have wondered this, but simply had no idea how to obtain such a goal.

Many of you have heard stories of old-time strongmen who performed almost unbelievable feats of hand and wrist strength, or local heroes who had a crushing grip, and let's not forget the lumberjacks of old who were able to chop wood with their mighty axes. With these inspiring stories, you may have decided to embark on your own program to obtain powerful hands. The only problem was, "How do I get started and what do I do?"

First you probably asked your high school football or baseball coach. He probably told you to squeeze a tennis ball every day. It wasn't long after this you realized that a tennis ball was made for tennis, not for squeezing. Next you probably went to a department store like K-Mart, or maybe your local sporting goods store, and bought what is known as your standard set of handgrippers. After a couple of weeks, you noticed you were jumping up on your reps and you were starting to feel a little bit macho, until your Aunt Martha grabbed the handgripper for the first time and closed it about ten times without even flinching.

From there you may have gone to your local gym and asked the gym owner for some ideas. After he scratched his head for a moment, he came up with the idea of basic wrist curls. That sounded great, you thought; after all, you remembered seeing Lou Ferrigno doing wrist curls in a magazine—and look at *his* powerful-looking forearms. But, once again, after a month or so of doing wrist curls you noticed only a slight gain in your hand strength. You may have noticed that your forearms looked bigger and stronger, which was good, but your goal of a powerful grip was only slightly closer, if any.

Once again we're back to the same question of, "How?" As a professional strongman who specializes in grip strength, I have tried and developed many exercises and new equipment. I have found that if you want an average grip you do average exercises, but if you want a great grip you do special exercises. Basically your goal of a powerful pair of hands and wrists has escaped you because of a lack of vision or know-how. The Holy Bible tells us that people perish because of a lack of vision.

In this book I will show you how to achieve your goals in lower arm strength, whatever they may be. I will guarantee you that if you follow these methods, you will be more than pleased with your development, whether you wish to be a professional strongman or a better rock climber, or hit a longer drive in golf. I will show you how to obtain a better grip without expensive equipment. I will also motivate you with challenges of old and new. I have found that motivation and positive momentum are keys to success in reaching any goal. Let's start gaining that momentum.

Chapter One

Champions of Yesterday and Today

Anyone who has ever read much on feats of hand strength has certainly been amazed by the records and feats of the strongmen of old. Whether it was one-hand deadlifting, card tearing, or bending horseshoes, the lower arms were always brought into use. On most of these strongmen you noticed a very muscular or sinewy look to their forearms. This was from years of training their lower arms.

Many of their feats of hand strength have remained as some of the greatest feats of all time. For instance, Hermann Goerner, who was easily one of the strongest men of all time, deadlifted with one hand a little over 700 pounds. Goerner also tore two packs of poker cards in half in exactly one second.

Batta, a French strongman known for great finger strength, used to tear a pack of poker cards in half using only the index finger and thumb of each hand. This required great muscle control of his fingers as well as strength, which can only be developed with proper training.

Thomas Inch of Britain was a great all-round strongman who also excelled in grip strength. Inch had a thick-handled dumbbell which was 2.47 inches thick at the shaft. The weight was 172 pounds. This may not sound that heavy for many good deadlifters; however for many,

many years, no one was able to lift this dumbbell even slightly off the ground. Only a handful of lifters have ever been able to break this dumbbell off the ground. It is now owned by a gentleman from Britain.

Many other strongmen have had challenge dumbbells which were rarely lifted. You have probably figured out by now that it is the thick handle that makes these dumbbells so difficult to lift. The regular dumbbell with a normal handle allows the lifter to wrap his hand completely around the bar. With the thick handle this cannot be done. This makes the lift a feat of hand strength instead of back and leg strength.

Many strongmen of old used bulky block weights for pinch grip lifting. I have written an entire chapter on block weights and their use.*

One-finger lifts were also very popular with early strongmen and also very dangerous. These lifts require much special training. Several strongmen have ruined the tendons in their fingers with these lifts. Later I will discuss one-finger lifts in more detail, but now let's look at some top performances. Warren Lincoln Travis was able to lift over 600 pounds with the middle finger of his right hand, and Jack Walsh once lifted a motorcycle around the weight of 570 pounds with the middle finger of his left hand. The great Joe Rollino of Brooklyn, New York, lifted 635 pounds with his middle finger. This spectacular lift was done at Coney Island at a bodyweight of only 175 pounds. When we talk about one-finger lifting, let us not forget Frank Phillip Brumbach who lifted 441 pounds with his little finger, or pinkie. These, or any traditional one-finger lifts, are performed by straddling the weight and placing your finger through a metal ring which is attached to the weight by chains or leather straps.

John Marx ("The Luxembourg Hercules") was a champion of grip strength. He was unmatched in lifting thick-handled dumbbells. He was asked to try and lift a challenge dumbbell of Noel, a French strongman. Noel's dumbbell had never been lifted before. Marx easily lifted it off the ground, then cleaned it and lifted it overhead with little difficulty. Marx was great in all feats of lower arm strength, but he was mainly known for his ability to break horseshoes. He was able to bend and break the largest and strongest horseshoes in all the land. In an exhibition he once bent and broke three large horseshoes in a little over three minutes. Later I will discuss horseshoe bending and breaking in more

---

*Editor's Note: John uses the term "block weight" for the end of a cast dumbbell, not a traditional block weight.

detail. It is a feat that requires tremendous power, not only in the arms and shoulders, but a great amount of lower arm strength as well. If there's a weak link in the hands, wrists, or forearms, the horseshoe will be the victor.

As you can see, there are many different ways the old-timers used to demonstrate their hand and wrist strength. The list could go on and on. I will mention one more contest that was popular years ago that most modern day strength athletes have probably never even heard of. The art of finger twisting and finger pulling was very popular. Vic Boff, the president of The Oldetime Barbell and Strongman Association, was never beaten in finger twisting. Vic beat many famous strength athletes in this game of finger strength. Vic is now in his upper 70's and retired from this test of fingers; however, until just a few years ago, he would still match his fingers against anyone who asked.

Very simply, finger twisting is done in this manner: Standing or seated you wrap any finger around your opponent's same finger (usually this is done with middle fingers), grasp tightly to his finger so that your fingers are hooked together, and now attempt to twist your wrist counter-clockwise, thus putting his finger in a bind. (Note: This is a very painful test and also has potential for finger injury.)

Now that we have looked at strongmen of old, let's look at some of the best of today.

Present Day Grip Masters

Strongmen of old give us general view of grip strength. As we explore modern day champions, we will begin to isolate the types of grip strength. For instance, crushing strength of grip is different than that of a viselike grip for holding onto objects. Or, the grip strength used for bending steel is different from the type of finger strength that is required for rock climbing. Our object is to develop a combination of all these types of lower arm strength to develop the ultimate grip.

One point I would like to make that seems to always be missed when it comes to lower arm strength is that large forearms do not mean one has a strong hand. I have found that hand strength, thumb strength, wrist strength, and forearm strength are all different and must be trained and treated differently. For example, you may see a bodybuilder with huge vein-choked forearms who has only an average grip. Once again, let's remember that the forearms are not the hands, and the hands are not the forearms. You may also find a farmer who has very thin forearms and a powerful grip. For example, Australian wheat farmer Bruce White pinch gripped 115 pounds on a smooth-plated weight with one hand, and he also pinch lifted 60 pounds using only the index finger and thumb of one hand. These lifts are among the best ever. My point here is that Bruce White weighs 148 pounds and has thin forearms and small wrists. The strength of the lower arms comes largely from the tendons and ligaments.

When one thinks of crushing strength of hand he usually thinks of crushing cans or squeezing someone's hand in a handshake until it turns to dust. There are several heavy-duty handgrippers on the market that are designed to develop a strong crushing grip as well as measure one's

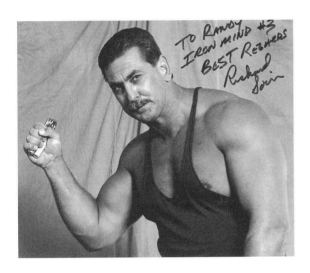

Richard Sorin mashing the #3 IronMind gripper. Photo courtesy of Richard Sorin.

crushing strength. IronMind® Enterprises, Inc. puts out a number of extra-strong high-grade grippers that are very quickly becoming the gauge for hand strength among strength athletes. The grippers range from Trainer to #1, #2, #3, and #4. The Trainer requires about 100 pounds of pressure to fully close; the #1 about 140 pounds; the #2 about 195 pounds; the #3 about 280 pounds; and the #4 about 365 pounds of pressure to close. The average person who lifts weights is unable to close even the #1.

As this book goes to press, only six people in the world have been able to fully close the #3: Richard Sorin of South Carolina was the first, I myself was second, and Tyce Saylor third. Ron Mazza (fourth), Eric Fitzsimmons (fifth), and Mark Smith (sixth) are all from Bollenbach's Gym in Monroe, New York. These grippers have been taken all over the world, and just about all of the top strength athletes from Olympic lifting to powerlifting to arm wrestling to Highland Games to strongman contests have tried. Many of the world's strongest men have bought the #3 gripper and trained with it for years, but have still been unable to close it. By the way, two 17-year-olds, Brian David and Robert Artmont, have closed the #2 gripper, which is pretty impressive considering their age.

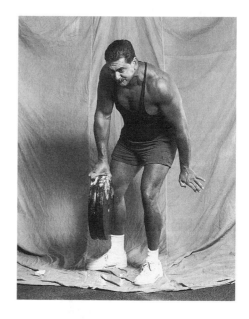

Richard Sorin pinch gripping two York 45-lb. plates. Photo courtesy of Richard Sorin.

Richard Sorin, in my opinion, has the strongest crushing grip in the world. He has been able to close the #3 gripper for years. What is truly amazing is that a couple of years ago at The Oldtime Barbell and Strongman dinner in New York, Richard actually closed the #3 gripper with two fingers. Now to give you some idea of how difficult this is, if you aren't familiar with these special handgrippers, the #3 gripper takes about 280 pounds of pressure to completely close, and the grippers that you can buy at a sporting goods store take about 30 pounds of pressure to close. Now imagine being able to close about nine or ten of these regular grippers at the same time with only two fingers. Sounds unbelievable, doesn't it? Well, Richard Sorin did it.

Richard's pinch gripping is truly amazing as well; he has pinch gripped a total of 123 pounds with one hand. This was done with two York 45-lb. plates held together and a bar through the middle to hold the extra plates. He can also take two York 45's, pinch grip them together, and then hand them from one hand to the other, showing his amazing gripping power in either hand. To gauge pinch gripping for one who has never tried it before, you must understand that it is probably the most deceptive-looking test of strength in the world. You grab two weight plates and turn them together so that the smooth part faces outward— this is the part the hand must grip. Now put your hand over the top of the plates with your fingers on one side and your thumb on the other, squeeze tightly as if trying to pinch the plates together, and lift them off the ground. If the weight you're lifting is too heavy, it will actually feel as if it is glued to the floor.

If you can lift two 25-lb. plates by the smooth side with one hand, you have a fairly good grip; most men cannot lift two 25-lb. plates in this manner. If you can lift two 35-lb. plates in a pinch grip, you have a very good grip; and if you are able to lift 90 pounds, or two 45-lb. plates in this fashion you have a world class pinch grip. After you try this type of lifting, you will realize just how strong Richard Sorin's grip really is. Besides Richard, here are a few other modern day strength athletes who excel in lower arm strength.

Dennis Rogers, a former arm wrestling world champion, now a professional strongman who has appeared on "David Letterman," "The Today Show," and "Regis and Kathie Lee," has a very good all-round grip. Dennis excels in all types of card tearing and phone book tearing. He is able to tear a pack of plastic-coated poker cards in half in a couple of seconds. He also tears the cards in half behind his back, no easy feat. The card tearing feat that Dennis has become somewhat famous for is his ability to tear cards with a set of thick oven mittens on his hands. This requires him to be able to grip the cards very tightly with just his fingertips; he also must be able to completely maintain his grip through-out the whole tearing feat. His fingertips must become like pliers to be able to perform this amazing feat of hand strength.

Dennis also is the world champion at tearing phone books. He tears the thickest books in the world *lengthwise*, making it more difficult. Most all phone book tearers, past and present, tear through the binding. The method Dennis uses is much harder, and he often wraps the books in duct tape (electrician's tape), making it even more difficult. Dennis also excels in bar bending and is a good pinch gripper.

Steve Sadicario ("The Mighty Stephan") is a very pleasant high-energy-packed strongman from New Jersey. "The Mighty Stephan" is a very good all-round performer who has several feats of hand and wrist strength worth mentioning. He is a very good card tearer, able to quickly tear in half and then quarter the cards with ease. He is able to tear license plates in his hands, a feat of strength seldom done. "The Mighty Stephan" excels in nail bending, able to bend very hard nails, and he often bends these nails while he sings in an opera voice, which is very entertaining.

The feat of lower arm strength that has always impressed me that "The Mighty Stephan" performs is chain breaking—yes, real chain breaking. "The Mighty Stephan" usually uses a No. 6 jack chain to break in his hands. This No. 6 gauge chain is a thick non-welded, twisted chain, which is hard to find any more. I have tested this chain by holding up an engine with it. I hoisted up 500 pounds and left to have lunch; when I came back the engine was still off the ground and the chain still holding. Later I added 100 pounds more, totaling 600 pounds, and then the chain started to slowly stretch and break. Now just imagine, it takes 600 pounds of pressure to break this chain. "The Mighty Stephan" is not breaking this chain with his legs or his back, but with his hands. He takes a short piece of chain and grasps it in his hands and then pulls and twists, breaking the chain. I have seen a lot of strength feats in my life, but this one is truly one of the greatest.

John Ottarski is a professional arm wrestler from North Carolina who trains his grip very hard in many interesting ways. He has been training for a long time now, well into his forties; he says he is still improving steadily. John has fairly large hands which he uses to the utmost. I met John a while back at his home. He took me out behind his house and showed me his tools of the grip trade he has in his storage shed. He likes to use thick-handled dumbbells to deadlift heavy weights. He lifted 153 pounds on a 2-1/2 inch shaft to demonstrate how he deadlifts. This shaft is a revolving shaft, making it much harder to lift, for when you grasp it to lift, it tries to spin out of your hand. This is very heavy lifting in this manner.

What I found even more interesting is that, instead of jumping up in weight as most people do, John uses the same weight. However, to keep improving on hand strength every workout, John simply adds a strand of tape to the bar, making it slightly thicker. This doesn't sound like much, but over a month's period of time you have a substantial difference. Little by little, one goes far. This may be the best way to improve on thick-handled lifting. There's no telling how thick that dumbbell handle is now.

Another similar exercise device John uses is a five-gallon bucket to do one-finger muscle outs. A muscle out is just like doing a front lateral raise, lifting from the ground to a position where your arm is held straight out in front of you. John usually hooks his little finger, or pinkie, through the metal loop and then lifts. He loads this bucket with ordinary sand. Every day he does this exercise, he adds one handful of sand. Here again, this is not enough weight to notice a difference with each workout; however, over a period of time, you have made a huge jump. We did not weigh the bucket of sand, but it was getting heavy for a muscle out with a little finger.

John's program of progressive gains is remarkable, and this way of training is virtually injury-free. Anyone who wants to improve and has the understanding of how long-term gains work could certainly learn a lot from John Ottarski.

Carl Braun is a heavyweight Highland Games champion. Carl is one of the best in the world with many records, particularly in the Scottish hammer. It is very likely Carl may in time be the world's greatest heavy weight athlete the Highland Games has ever seen. Carl will be quick to point out that in the heavy weight events like the 56-lb. weight toss for height or distance or in the hammer throw, the grip is a key element, and if the grip is not strong the throw will be poor. Carl does not normally practice feats of hand strength. However, through years of training for the Highland Games, throwing hammers and tossing cabers, he has developed very strong hands as well as very tough hands.

Tyce Saylor is a strength athlete from California who has a unique training program and was the third person to completely close the #3 IronMind gripper. I understand he has recently started competing in the Highland Games. More interesting when it comes to hand strength is that Tyce says he was able to close the #3 gripper because he has been doing an exercise in which he grasps a 100-lb. dumbbell in each hand and walks a certain distance with these heavy weights. If he tires, he sets the weights down very briefly then grabs them again and continues. Since Tyce has closed the #3 gripper, we will certainly have respect for his method, and we will probably see a lot of would-be gripmasters out carrying weights for distance.

Sonny Upole is a close friend of mine who often helps me with my strongman programs. Sonny was a good powerlifter. He is a powerful man with a great grip. He has never trained his grip for strength in the normal way. All his life, Sonny has worked hard splitting wood and doing manual labor. Sonny had never heard of the IronMind grippers when I showed them to him. He looked at them, grabbed the #2, and with no hesitation closed it completely. What makes this so amazing is that I have never heard of anyone closing the #2 gripper without training on them for a while. He closed it so easily it was almost comical, and remember, he does no special grip training at all. This says a lot for hard manual labor, doesn't it?*

Al Wahlman is an interesting man from the Pacific Northwest. Al is an amateur strongman who does a handful of strength acts a year. He has a fine grip as well as a lot of overall strength. He does phone book tearing, nail bending, and many other fine strength feats.

Al has two feats of hand strength that deserve special mention. First we will discuss his ability to break thick glasses with his fingertips. Al sets several very thick milk or drinking glasses on the table and puts only his fingertips over the lip of a glass and squeezes. The glass breaks at the very top under Al's great finger strength. At first glance this might not sound very hard to perform; however, these thick glasses are very hard to break with just straight pressure. Everyone thinks of how easily glass breaks when you drop it, but breaking it with just straight pressure is another thing. Also, Al does this with just his fingertips, not his whole hand.

If you decide to try this feat, be careful not to cut yourself. You may want to use a thin glove for protection. Also, be careful not to hyperextend your thumb when you grasp the top of the glass. This problem sometimes occurs with certain types of pinch gripping, when the thumb is bent back slightly under the pressure exerted on the object being gripped. This generally happens when a pinch grip with the fingertips is being performed. We will discuss this more in the chapter about block weights. After you try to break a thick glass in this manner, you will probably gain respect for this deceptive feat.

Al's other feat I will mention may sound impossible to perform, but it is legitimate and truly performed by Al. Al uses a regular pair of pliers that are still in the package, to show that the pliers have not been tampered with. Al removes the pliers from the package and places a nut or several coins between the prongs of the pliers, causing the handles to spread a couple of inches apart. Now Al grasps the handles in his right hand and places his left hand over his right hand and squeezes with all his might. Suddenly the pliers break at the handles with a mighty snap.

*Editor's Note: I've personally watched Cleve Dean, the phenomenal superheavyweight arm wrestler, absolutely mash a #2 gripper on sight. Cleve, a former farmer, has also done a lot of manual labor.

This has always amazed Al's audiences. Al always lets anyone in the audience try to break the pliers first; no one has. He has done this feat with all types and name brands of pliers including the famous Craftsman pliers. This is truly one of the greatest feats of lower arm strength ever performed.

Well, we have looked at some old-time strength stars and their feats and also some modern day people, some known professionals and some unknown people who deserved special mention. Now it's time to get you started on the road to grip greatness.

Chapter Two

Grip Strength — What is It?

Let's now take a closer look at the different types of grip strength and power, as well as the ways to acquire it.

First of all, when someone thinks of grip strength, he generally thinks of crushing force or simply the force one is able to squeeze in the handshake position, or the force one can generate squeezing a handgripper. The fact is that this is only one type of hand strength. Although this type of gripping power certainly should not be over-looked, it is not any more important than a number of other hand strengths.

Individual finger strength is a tremendous asset in any sport or in any activity. A rock climber certainly understands the importance of strength in all the fingers. Also, the martial artist must have this type of fingertip strength for any type of gouging or clawing technique.

We also must develop a strong set of thumbs if we are truly serious about developing a powerful set of hands. Many men who have a strong crushing or squeezing grip have little strength when it comes to any type of pinch gripping. You may also find that some world-class deadlifters, who can hold onto the bar with incredible poundages, may only have an average pinch grip. The reason for this is the simple fact that their thumbs are not developed like the rest of their hands.

Also, the hand strength used to open the hand is important and should not be overlooked if you are serious about developing overall hand strength. You will find that if you develop the different kinds of grip strength, each one will help you gain strength with the others. When you desire to develop grip strength for a certain sport or activity, you must research the kind of hand strength you need to develop.

You first need to examine the way your hand is shaped for your desired movement. You must see how wide your hand is opened for the object you are grasping or squeezing. For instance, if you are trying to hold onto the bar for a heavy deadlift, you will notice that your hand is almost completely closed. Now, studying your hand in this position, you will notice that the grip used in the deadlift position is completely different from the hand position used in a pinch grip position. Also, the hand position used in pinch gripping a narrow object is much different from the hand position used to grasp a wide object. Once again, if you are serious about developing the type of strength needed for your goal, you need to examine the shape your hand will be in and also the amount your hand is opened.

As we mentioned above, the best program for lower arm strength is a total grip program, emphasizing all the different kinds of gripping power and also the different positions of the hand opening and closing. I suggest that many different exercises be used in your program, with extra attention to the movements that will especially assist you in reaching your desired goal. You are probably wondering by now, "How am I going to work all this in my busy schedule?"

I receive many calls and letters from all different types of athletes wanting to know how to develop the type of hand strength they need for their desired sport. Often a martial artist who is training in a kung fu animal style, like eagle claw or praying mantis, calls me for ideas to enhance his grip for clawing and grasping techniques. In these types of kung fu, the strength of the fingers is of the utmost importance. Some of the trainees tell me that they train by squeezing handgrippers. Although squeezing heavy handgrippers will help develop their hand strength, the grippers are probably the least helpful method for their desired goal.

The position the hand is in for the techniques used in the eagle claw or the praying mantis methods are much different from the position the hand is in when squeezing a handgripper. For the eagle claw, the hand is opened to grasp and claw with the fingers, with a large emphasis put on the thumb. An ancient method used to develop strength of hand for kung fu clawing techniques is bag catching. We will look closely at this exercise in Chapter 3., Building Your Crushing Grip.

I have also had many letters and calls from rodeo professionals who want to obtain a stronger grip for bull or bronco riding. Their type of gripping requires them to grasp a medium-sized rope and to hang on tightly for the ride. This also requires an extremely strong wrist, and much attention needs to be placed on the entire lower arm. This type of grip strength is similar to heavy deadlifting; however, the training required for rodeo and the stress put on the hand and wrist for rodeo are much different from heavy deadlifting.

Professional arm wrestling is another sport that emphasizes hand strength. Actually arm wrestling could be called hand wrestling. Years ago arm wrestling was much different from the modern day advanced techniques. In those days, arm wrestlers simply pulled as hard as they could, attempting to pin their opponents to the table. Also, all the pressure was lateral or side pressure.

The modern day professional uses techniques so advanced that a person not knowing the techniques, no matter how strong, could walk into a professional arm wrestling meet and not have a chance of winning against an experienced professional. These modern day techniques emphasize hand strength in many different ways. If you can overpower your opponent's hand, the rest of his arm will follow. Most serious arm wrestlers train by doing barbell curls and wrist curls, just like the old-time arm wrestlers. However, much of their training consists of special grip training that will help them develop their arm wrestling techniques for these modern times.

The Thumb

The thumb is of the utmost importance when it comes to grip strength, and it is often overlooked. Many athletes wonder why they lack the grip strength they desire. In many cases it is because they have not developed their thumbs. As many of you have probably learned, strong thumbs are required for pinch gripping, as well as lifting thick-handled dumbbells. By building up your thumb strength you will also build your crushing strength. The reason for this is because your whole hand works in unison.

I have included many styles of lifting in the exercise section which will help strengthen your thumbs. All types of pinch gripping will strengthen your thumbs. Whether you are pinch gripping or training your thumbs on IronMind's Titan's Telegraph Key, it is important to understand how the thumb works. While the thumbs are potentially very strong, they can be easily strained if you haven't been training them.

They can be strained by overtraining or they can also be injured by hyperextending them.

Hyperextending your thumbs simply means trying to grasp something which is too wide for your hand to grip. This stretches the thumb joints past their limits. I can tell you from experience that a strained thumb isn't a lot of fun. About five years ago, a friend of mine made me a large block of steel that he thought would help strengthen my grip. He had attached a loading pin to the bottom so that I could add as much weight as I wanted. I used this block of steel to pinch grip. I immediately noticed that the block was hard to lift because it was so wide. It was hard for my hand to span the top of the block. I used this block for a few workouts. After about a week I decided to go up to a higher weight. As a result, I strained the thumb on my left hand. I realized the whole time that the block was too wide, but I went ahead and kept using it anyway. The pain in my thumb lasted for about five months. This

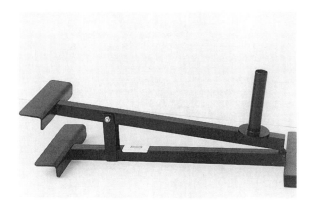

IronMind's Titan's Telegraph Key works your individual fingers and thumb. While it's typically used on a table, John Brookfield pioneered training on it while sitting in a recliner, which he says puts it in a perfect position! Photo by Randall J. Strossen, Ph.D.

was five years ago and occasionally I can still feel the spot in my thumb joint when I'm training my grip.

When you start training your thumbs, be careful not to strain your thumb or grasp something so wide that your thumb joint is being stretched. Do not let this scare you off from training your thumbs. It is even very productive for your grip to pinch grip wide objects. Like anything, you must use common sense. You can tell the minute you grab an object if it is too wide for your hand or not. Just train smart and consistently and you will continue to improve. Always remember that your thumbs are made for something other than twiddling.

While we have discussed only a few kinds of grip strength, there are many kinds used for many different sports and activities. We could go on and on with a huge list of different sports and the importance of the lower arms in these sports, but all the knowledge in the world won't help us if we don't put it in action.

In the following chapter we will look at many different exercises. These exercises cover all kinds of lower arm strength for everything from sports to different kinds of strength feats. I will explain many exercises for each type of lower arm strength. There are exercises designed for limited space that can be done in a small city apartment; and there are also exercises that can be done in the most primitive, most remote areas on earth, using nothing but natural surroundings.

Chapter Three

Building Your Crushing Grip

In this chapter we will look at some different ways to develop crushing strength in the hands. As we said before, when most people wish to gain strength in the hands, they think of crushing force.

The special handgrippers on the market, like the IronMind Captains of Crush Grippers™ and also the Ivanko Super Gripper are very good. These types of grippers are usually the only thing people think of when it comes to developing crushing strength in the hands, but there are actually many, many more. Let's look at a few other great exercises to help your crushing grip. I will also show you how to do them and what material is required.

Wire Cutting

A great way to build a powerful handshake and crushing force in your grip is cutting wires with wire cutters. I know what you're thinking. Your Uncle Melvin is an electrician and he cuts wire all the time and his grip isn't all that great. If his grip isn't that great, it is because electricians and other professionals who cut a lot of wire always use a pair of wire cutters that are much bigger than the wires they are cutting. In other words, they use wire cutters that can easily cut through the wire with little effort.

In our case, we are going to use a pair of wire cutters that make it difficult to cut the wire. I have cut a lot of wire in my day, some on fences working on a job, but I have cut even more wire while training my grip. I can also tell you that cutting wire in this fashion will toughen up your hands. To have a really strong grip which can be used for all purposes, you need tough hands.

All you need to get started is a pair of wire cutters. They would be best if they are on the small side. If you don't own a pair, you can purchase a pair at a hardware store for a few dollars. If you live on a farm or in the country, you can easily find some wire, old or new, you can use. If you live in the city, you can purchase some wire at a store. It won't be very expensive and the wire will go a long way the way we are going to use it. The best wire to use is regular fence wire that you see around most farms. This size wire has the right strength and thickness to give your grip a workout.

After you have your wire and your wire cutters, all you have to do is find the end of the wire and cut the wire inch by inch with the wire cutters. I usually cut it off about an inch at a time. You can even cut off a little less than an inch if you would like. As you can see, a little wire goes a long way in this fashion. If you are outside, you can let the wire pieces you cut off fall on the ground, or also in a bucket, if you desire. This will keep them from getting in your yard. If you are indoors, you will need to let them fall into a bucket or can. Always face the end of the wire which you are cutting toward or over the bucket so it will fall into the bucket. This will also keep the piece from hitting you.

You will want to change hands to get an equal workout. You will notice that this exercise really works the hands when a wire cutter is used that requires you to really squeeze the wire to cut it. If you have a pair of cutters that easily cuts the wire and you can't find another pair, you may want to overlap the wire so that you are cutting off two pieces together. This will give you the same effect. As you get stronger, you can get even thicker wire or a smaller pair of cutters. You can also start cutting the wire with only three or two fingers. Give this exercise a try; it will really help your crushing grip and toughen up your hands.

Plier Lifting

Another great way to strengthen the crushing force of your hand is by lifting things with pliers. I discovered this method a few years ago when I was just playing around. All you need is a pair of pliers—any pliers will do. Also you will need a five-gallon bucket. You will need to place some type of weight in the bucket—dirt, rocks, sand, weight plates, or even water if you have a lid on the bucket to keep the water from splashing out. Once you have the bucket weighted, take a piece of leather from an old belt or wherever you can find one. Put the piece of

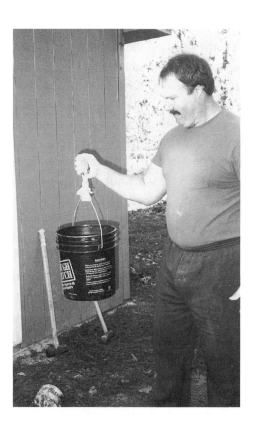

John demonstrates plier lifting with a bucket. Photo by Steve Jeck.

leather underneath the handle of the bucket. Now bring the two ends of the leather together over the top of the handle. The leather is basically making a loop or a ring through the handle of the bucket.

Now from here, all you do is grasp the pliers with the handles upward and the clamp facing downward. Grip the leather tightly with the pliers. Now lift the bucket off the ground with the pliers. You will notice that you must maintain a very tight grip on the handles of the pliers. The weight pulling down on the pliers is constantly trying to break your grip.

A good exercise after you lift the bucket with the pliers is hammer curls. This lifting up and down motion will make it even harder to keep a tight grip on the leather with the pliers. You can see how long you can hold the weight off the ground or you can see how much weight you can lift in this manner.

Be sure to use a fairly thick piece of leather so that it won't break under the strain. If you use a cloth instead of leather, be sure that the cloth is very strong.

Another way to do plier lifts is to use a regular barbell. Take two pieces of leather or heavy cloth and loop them under the bar, so that the weight will be equally balanced. You can now take two pairs of pliers and clamp one pair onto one piece of leather and the other pair onto the other piece. You can now perform deadlifts or hammer curls. Lifting with pliers is very challenging as well as rewarding. A tremendous crushing grip can be developed by lifting weight with pliers.

Double Hammer Squeeze

Another great crushing force exercise can be done with two sledge hammers. The hammers should be of normal length. Normal length is usually 36 inches from the top of the hammer to the end of the handle. Most men who have pretty good grips can probably use two eight-pound hammers. If you don't train your grip regularly, you may need to start with two six-pound hammers.

Once you have your hammers and are ready to start, I would suggest doing this exercise outside. If it's cold or raining and you decide to do it inside, be sure to have plenty of room. To start, lay both sledge hammers on the ground. The ends of the handles should meet each other, with the heads of the hammers going in opposite directions. Simply put, if your hammers were a clock, one hammer head would be at 12 o'clock and the other hammer head would be at six o'clock (see photos next page).

Once your hammers are in this position, overlap the ends of the handles about four inches. It can vary a little bit depending on your hand size, but basically you want to overlap the handles about the width of your hand. If you overlap the handles too much, it will make the exercise too easy; and if you overlap the handles much less than the width of your hand, you will have a hard time getting any kind of grip on the handles. You may want to mark it with tape once you find the right spot. Now reach down and grab the overlapped handles and lift the hammers off the ground using only one hand. You will quickly notice that this has the same effect as holding a heavy-duty gripper closed.

If you figure out the weight at the ends of the hammer with the length of the handles, you will find out you have a great amount of

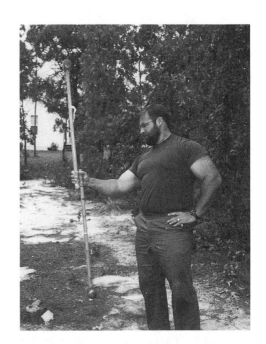

Steve Jeck shows the double hammer squeeze both in the frontal raise (above right), and horizontal position (below right). Photos by John Brookfield.

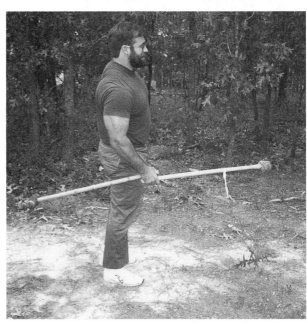

resistance trying to open your hand. You can either hold onto the hammers as long as you can, or you can even lift the hammers off the ground and do a frontal raise with them. At one time I used to take the hammers from the frontal raise and then lift them over my head like a clean and press. Be very careful if you try this. The hammers can easily slip, and also your grip position will change: When you're holding the hammers off the ground in the deadlift position, most of the pressure is on the index and forefinger; but when the hammers are turned over or cleaned to your shoulder, all the pressure is on your two smaller fingers. Be sure and do equal training with each hand.

As you get stronger, you can of course hold the hammers longer. If you decide to use more weight, you can purchase heavier hammers or, to save on expense, you can simply weld a piece of steel on the heads of the hammers so you can put small weight plates on top. If you don't have plates, a brick with holes can be added as well. Try this hammer lift and you will get the hand workout of your life.

Grip Machine

Another great way to help build a superb crushing grip is the grip machine. The grip machine is a steel plate-loading piece of equipment that you can squeeze with one or two hands. You can use as little or as much weight as you would like (see photo). You can also change the distance between the bars you are squeezing together. If you have a small hand, you may wish to put a small weight plate or a piece of wood at the bottom. IronMind® Enterprises, Inc. sells great grip machines for a reasonable price.

If you have access to some scrap steel and you know a good welder who is not too expensive, you can also make your own. It would take a small book in itself for me to explain to you how to make one from start to finish; however, if you look at the picture of the grip machine, you can easily figure out how it works and how to make one. I had a friend of mine weld one for me. On mine I left out the bar on the bottom that holds the weight plates. Instead, I put a steel tray. I chose the tray so I could use a variety of objects for weight, instead of just plates. By doing this, I can use concrete blocks, buckets of sand, large rocks or, of course, weight plates. If you make your own, I suggest using the tray, especially if you don't own a lot of weights.

In choosing the right poundage to begin with, you will have to experiment. Some like to do a lot of repetitions for endurance and some like to train heavy for power. If you're training one hand at a time, you will probably want to start out with a weight of about 50 pounds to get the feel of the exercise. It is very important not to pull up or deadlift the weight. Be sure to just squeeze the bars together. While it is good to continually try to use heavier poundages to build up your crushing strength, many people lose good form by slightly deadlifting the bottom bar as they try to reach their maximum poundage.

I have found that by doing a lot of repetitions you can actually gain forearm size very quickly. On the other hand, you can gain tremendous finger strength by very heavy training. This makes the grip machine a highly effective tool.

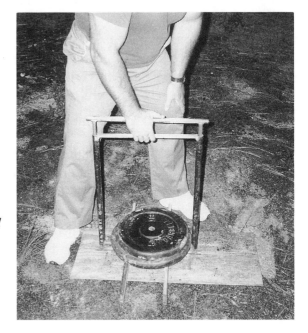

Steve Jeck demonstrates John's grip machine, which can be loaded with bricks, etc. if you're short on barbell plates. Photo by John Brookfield.

Bag Catching

I have included bag catching in this section because, if it is done properly, it will enhance your crushing strength, as well as help you develop a very explosive grip. I do not include bag catching as a regular part of my training although I use it occasionally to cross-train my grip. Bag catching is especially good for martial artists and rock climbers. It is an exercise that can be done anywhere.

All you need is a money or currency bag. You can find a money bag at your local bank. They will usually give you one free or sell you one for very little. Now you need to fill the bag with steel shot. At the local gun shop you can purchase steel shot. It's a little expensive at times. In my bag I use very small screws that I purchased at the hardware store. They work just as well and were much cheaper. The choice is yours.

Load your currency bag full of the metal. Load it tightly, but not to where it is hard to close up the zipper. After you close the bag, take some duct tape and tape over the entire bag, especially over the zipper. This will reinforce the bag so it will last. Now we are ready to start. Take the bag in one hand and toss it up in the air about head high; now snatch it out of the air with the other hand. Repeat this by tossing it with *that* hand and grabbing it with the first hand. Continue this until you're tired. Always be sure to grab the bag the same amount of times with each hand.

You will notice that the bag is not very heavy. The weight of the bag is not the object of this exercise. The object is to grab the bag as quickly and explosively as possible. Each time you grab the bag, grab it as if you were trying to tear it apart—the same way an eagle uses its talons to grab its prey. Bag catching is great for developing the tendons of your fingers and explosive power in your lower arms.

Heavy-duty Handgrippers

Of all the phone calls I receive from people wanting to develop a stronger grip, most athletes are interested in the heavy-duty grippers. They either want to know how often they should use them, or how many repetitions they should do to get the most out of their training. First of all, right now I don't use the grippers myself on a regular basis. However, I can tell you that they are very helpful for developing a powerful crushing grip. I also feel that they are only a part of what is required to develop a great overall grip, a grip that can be used for all situations, from sports to any kind of lifting or any kind of daily activity whatsoever.

The reason for this is that when you are using heavy-duty handgrippers, the thumb is not being used. The thumb is almost always the weakest link in an athlete's grip. The reason I'm talking about the thumb in the section about handgrippers is that I have met many, many strength athletes who think all they have to do to develop a great grip is to use heavy-duty grippers.

Now, let's get back to the grippers. I feel that most people whose hands are already in good condition can profit from using the IronMind grippers or the Ivanko Super Gripper three times a week. Remember that you know your own body better than anyone else. So, if you feel that three times a week is too much, or that it isn't enough, go with what works for you. You have probably heard that you can work your forearms and hands every day. With light or endurance training this may be so. However, with the heavy-duty grippers, you will find that squeezing them as hard as it takes to close them will literally wear your hand out if you don't rest a day between workouts. Anyone who uses them will

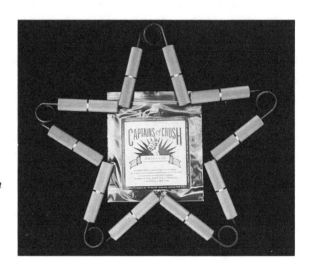

IronMind's Captains of Crush Grippers™, the established star in their field. Photo by Randall J. Strossen, Ph.D.

find out that they are nearly impossible to put down, especially when you have a gripper that you can't completely close. It always seems that you just keep trying and trying. This, of course, overtrains your hand. It is very good to be energetic about your training, but be careful about falling into this try-and-try-again category. Just train sensibly, and you will make more consistent progress.

As far as how many sets and repetitions you should do, you can basically use the same principle as with any other type of resistance training, if you're trying to maximize your crushing grip. You should do about five sets with each hand. Always do a warm-up or light set to get your circulation going, then go on to a few heavy sets of around four or five repetitions. Since the IronMind grippers have only a few different strengths, you may have to do more repetitions on a lighter gripper to work up to the next gripper. This will be just as productive. If, for instance, you can do 20 repetitions on the #1 gripper, and only one repetition on the #2, I would suggest doing about 10 reps on the #1 to warm up and then trying to close the #2 gripper as many times as you can for three or four sets. After this, I would finish by closing the #1 as many times as I could.

If you are patient and stick to a program like this, you will steadily progress. You may also find it helpful as you get stronger to do a set or two closing one of the easier grippers with only your index and middle fingers. If this is a little too difficult, try a set with only three fingers. Heavy-duty grippers will enhance your crushing grip as well as your confidence.

Chapter Four

Building Your Pinch Grip

In this chapter we will discuss many different ways to pinch grip. In my opinion, pinch gripping is of vital importance in developing a powerful grip. It is much neglected by many athletes, even those who train their grips regularly. The pinch grip is a great way to develop thumb strength. I must stress again that thumb strength comes into play much more than most people realize. Any type of grasping thick objects brings into play your thumb strength.

It is also very important to realize the different types of pinch gripping. For instance, the hand is opened different widths depending on how wide the object is that you are pinch gripping. For example, your hand is opened twice as wide gripping a large block weight than it is pinch gripping a regular weight plate. If you can invest the time, I would try to pinch grip two or three different-sized objects. This will give you a good overall grip. However, I realize as much as anyone that time is limited and you may not have enough time to invest in this type of training. If this is your case, look at your reason for training your grip and decide what type of pinch gripping will be the most productive for your individual case. Some sports or activities require more strength with your hand wide open and some require strength with your hand opened less.

Wide Grip Pinch Gripping

As far as pinch gripping wide objects, the block weights described in Chapter 5, Training With Block Weights, are the best for wide grip training. Of course the heavier the block weight, the wider the grip; all the block weights described are sufficient to train the hand in this wide grip technique. I feel that using a wide grip is the most profitable for myself. When I'm strong in the wide grip pinch lift, my grip is at its strongest for overall purposes. Follow the exercises in the chapter on block weights to improve your wide grip strength.

There, of course, are other objects to lift in this fashion. I will very briefly touch on a couple. Anvil lifting is a great way to develop strength in many ways. Of course, lifting an anvil by the horn is a great way to build a good grip; however, right now let's concentrate on pinch gripping the anvil by grasping it over the top. This will create a wide grip style. If you have an anvil around 50 lbs. it will be just about right for the average man who has done some hand training. An anvil of 70 to 80 lbs. will take a very strong-handed man to lift with a pinch grip. Richard Sorin has lifted an anvil weighing 100 lbs. in this fashion. This is absolutely incredible. Also, remember that if you have access to an anvil around 100 lbs. or a little more, you can train by doing a two-handed lift. You can also save on time by training this way. If you lift this way, be sure you lift heavy enough to help you achieve your goal.

I realize that most of you don't have access to an anvil for lifting. Another object you can perform wide grip lifting with is a wide wooden timber. You can find these timbers in any lumber yard. If the timber you use is too heavy, all you have to do is cut the timber to the right size for you to lift. I like a longer wooden timber so I can perform exercises using both hands. It is amazing how useful these timbers can be. I like to perform a whole program of exercises using the timber. Just pinch grip it with both hands and you are ready to perform bent-over rows, clean and jerks, deadlifts, and even curls. Just imagine how much your grip will develop if you perform these exercises using a pinch grip. You will also find that a timber like this is not very expensive. You may also be able to find an old one lying around a farm somewhere that you might be able to get free.

Be careful when pinch gripping any kind of wooden objects. You can pick up large splinters if you're not careful. You may also want to blunt the edge of the timber so it won't be so sharp. Some of these types of exercises may seem a little strange. However, always remember if you do regular exercises you will develop a regular grip. So it goes without saying that if you want a unique type of grip strength, you will need to perform unique exercises for your grip.

I will very briefly touch on one more exercise that will develop wide grip hand strength. If you have weight plates at home, or if you train at a gym, you can take about four 10-lb. discs and put them together and pinch grip them. If your hands and wrists are strong enough, you can perform curls with them. One-arm rows are also a great grip developer. You can probably find a lot of other objects that can be pinch gripped in the same fashion as the exercises we have mentioned.

Regular Grip Pinch Gripping

As for regular width pinch gripping, weight plates are a favorite and excellent way to develop strong thumbs and fingers. If you haven't done much pinch gripping, it may feel hard at first. Start with two 25-lb. plates. Make sure you turn the plates together, so that the smooth sides of the plates are facing outward and the lip or overhang of the plates is facing inward. Now all you have to do is grasp the plates over the top with your fingers on one side and your thumb on the other side, squeeze tightly and lift. When pinch gripping metal, you will find it helpful to use lifting chalk or some type of rosin to keep the surface dry and free of moisture.

A person starting out who has a reasonable amount of hand strength can probably lift two 25-lb. plates. If this is too much, you may want to use two or three 10-lb. plates. As you progress, you can run a bar or rod through the holes of the plates and add smaller plates as you get stronger. If you have a really good grip, you may be able to use two 35-lb. plates. If you can pinch grip two York 45-lb. plates by the smooth side with one hand, you are a world class pinch gripper. There are only a few people in the world who can perform this feat of hand strength, to give you some idea of the potential of this lift. There have been only about five or six men throughout history who have been able to pinch grip 100 lbs. or more with one hand.

After you find a weight you can pinch grip comfortably, you can then swing the weight to make it more difficult to hang onto. You can also pass it from hand to hand, or even pass it from one hand to the other behind your back. You can, of course, hold it with one hand as long as you can, or even lift the weight with two fingers as you improve. I have named a few exercises to help you with pinch gripping. There are many more that can be done—it's up to you.

I will mention one exercise to beware of. The clean is a very dangerous exercise to perform while pinch gripping plates. There have been a few men who have done cleans occasionally while pinch gripping two plates together; however, it is extremely dangerous for more reasons than one. First, it puts a tremendous strain on the wrist. Second, the plates are also prone to pull apart when they get to shoulder level. This, of course, could cause them to hit you in the shoulder. Last but not least, you will notice that the plates are very close to your face when you are cleaning them to your shoulder. If they slide at all when they are in that position, they can cause a very toothy experience. Cleaning block weights while pinch gripping is of great benefit, but two plates held together is a little too risky.

Another great way to train your pinch grip with a medium or normal grip is pinch gripping boards together. If you take a couple of 2" x 4"s and place them together and add a little, you have a great tool for building a mighty grip. It is probably best to cut your boards to about four feet in length. To add weight you can either take a couple of buckets and hang the handles over the ends of the two boards, or you can tie a couple of ropes attached to weight plates at the ends of the boards. This way you can use as much or as little weight in the buckets or with the plates as you like. You can perform deadlifts, rows, or even upright rows. Once again, some of these exercises may seem a little primitive or crude; however, they are the types of exercises that will build your grip to the standards that you desire.

Earlier we mentioned pinch gripping using a narrow grip or a grip where your hand is only slightly open. The same exercises that we just talked about with two boards can be performed using just one board. You can use one 2" x 4" or even a thinner board. Few people train their grip with such a thin object. This type of exercise will give your grip a great advantage.

Another way to train a close grip is to have a piece of steel about the size of a 50-cent piece welded to a block weight or other heavy piece of steel. You can try to lift this object using whatever grip you can get on the small piece of steel. It will be extremely challenging. Professional arm wrestler John Ottarski drilled a hole in a 50-cent piece and then ran a wire through the hole and tied the wire to a five-gallon bucket. John uses this to pinch grip. He can only grasp the coin with his thumb and forefinger. I mentioned John's training methods in Chapter 1. John lifts the coin and the bucket every day, adding a handful of sand to the bucket each day.

In the late 1800s there was a strongman who could lift 28 lbs. grasping a knitting needle with his thumb and forefinger. Imagine pinch gripping 28 lbs. with a thumb and forefinger, holding onto a thin, slick knitting needle. This certain strongman performed this feat for years, offering a wager to anyone who could duplicate the feat. His money was pretty safe.

There was also a Swiss dentist who used to pull teeth with his fingers. He would grab the tooth which needed to be extracted and wiggle and pull on it with his thumb and forefinger until it came out. This, of course, is a great feat of finger strength, but it is even more difficult than most people realize because of the moisture inside the mouth, which makes the tooth harder to hang onto. There were also some Japanese dentists who trained their fingers to pull teeth in the same manner. They developed this great finger strength by driving small pieces of wood into a board. They would then pull the pieces of wood out of the board with just their thumb and forefinger. This exercise is very similar to the technique which they used to pull teeth with their fingers.

I trained my fingers in a very similar manner just to try their method. I took a wooden plank about two inches thick and hammered cut nails down into the wood. I would then grasp the top of the nail with my thumb and forefinger and pull and twist until it came out. This type of gripping really works the hand muscles. I used to practice this method for about 15 minutes at a time. I would hammer three or four pieces of steel or cut nails into the plank and then pull them out one after the other. After I pulled them all out I would hammer them back into the wood and repeat the process over and over.

If you decide to try this type of training, I would suggest using pieces of steel instead of pieces of wood. The steel won't break like the wood and the steel will also be easier to hammer into the wooden plank. You can purchase a few cut nails from the hardware store and then cut off the top or the head of the nail. You will then have a piece of steel very similar in size to a tooth. Many people probably haven't heard of cut nails before. If you ask at a hardware store they will show you the cut nails you will need. They have the shape of a golf tee with a thinner head. You can use any small chunk of steel as well. You will probably want to file any burrs or sharp edges off the steel so it won't cut your fingers.

Mr. Pinch-O-Grip

Mr. Pinch-O-Grip is a little invention I came up with one day when I was lifting a timber with a pinch grip. It is extremely easy to put together. All you need is a 2" x 12" lumber about 30 inches long or even a little longer. You will also need two pieces of 2" x 4" about 10 inches long. Now take your pieces of 2" x 4" and place one at each end of your 2" x 12". Nail the 2" x 4"s into the 2" x 12" with the long four-inch piece sticking up and the two-inch piece nailed flat into the 2" x 12". If this is confusing, look at the photo closely to understand. Place several

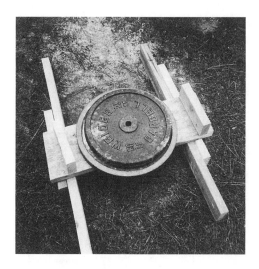

Mr. Pinch-O-Grip, loaded with weight plates and ready for use. Photo by Steve Jeck.

nails in each end to make the device durable enough to withstand the weight.

Now that you've built your Mr. Pinch-O-Grip, you're ready to go lifting. The reason we made the platform 30 inches long is so you can place Olympic barbell plates on the platform between the 2" x 4"s. You can also place concrete blocks on the platform. Now you will be performing a two-handed deadlift using the 2" x 4"s to pinch grip. This piece of equipment is well worth the effort to make. You can use as little or as much weight as you would like. You can have a great gripping contest with this device. I would say that 200 lbs. in this lift is a very good lift. You may want to elevate the platform by placing blocks under each end of your Mr. Pinch-O-Grip. This will make it easier on your back to deadlift, as well as protect your feet if your grip slips while you are lifting.

Everywhere I take this invention people are always very interested in it. They usually end up making their own. Lifting with Mr. Pinch-O-Grip will really develop your grip to new heights. I like to start out with a warm-up set and then work up to heavier and heavier weights with each set. Sometimes I even lift to my maximum on this lift. Be sure to warm up your fingers before trying to lift heavy on this exercise.

Axe Head Lifting

As you can see, there are many, many ways to develop and challenge your grip. Another way I like to pinch grip is to drive an axe head into a log. Drive the axe head deep enough that it won't slip out and be sure to leave enough out to grip. The axe head will make a perfect object to

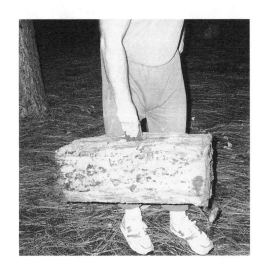

John walks a stout log by pinch gripping an axe head embedded in it. Photo by Steve Jeck.

pinch grip (see photo). I used to have a 60-lb. piece of pine that I would drive an axe head into, then pinch grip it with one hand and walk as far as I could before dropping it. I also used to drive two axe heads into a log that weighed about 200 lbs. and deadlift the log. It was a real challenge hanging onto this kind of weight with two slick axe heads. If you live in the country or a rural area, you can really have fun with this one.

My axe heads don't have the wooden handles on them, but you can do these lifts just as easily with the handles left on. You can drive a regular wedge into the log as well. This is the type of wedge used to split wood. You can lift more weight with the wedge than with the axe head because the wedge is tapered, allowing you to get a better grip on it. This type of gripping contest would be great for a lumberjack festival.

Rope Climbing

Rope climbing is a very ancient way to develop strength. Few people practice rope climbing anymore. If you can find a rope climber, you will notice that they always have a well-developed pair of forearms and a strong grip. Rope climbing stresses the lower arms to the utmost. There are a handful of arm wrestlers that practice rope climbing to develop their forearms, hands, and wrists.

One very important thing to remember is that the more you weigh, the harder rope climbing becomes. This is why rope climbing is practiced by small men. For instance, a gymnast who is muscular and light in weight who rope climbs is merely toning his body. Not that rope climbing is not productive for a lighter person because it will still help develop the hands and arms, but just think of the power workout a person weighing 200 lbs. or more will get. If a man weighing 250 lbs. can rope climb, he will develop world class strength in his upper and lower arms. I urge larger athletes to practice this. It is extremely hard work at first, but think of the benefits.

I understand that most people don't have access to a climbing rope. If you do, that's great; but if not, here's a way you can get the same benefits. Purchase a short piece of rope from the hardware. The rope should be about three feet long. Also be sure to buy the thickest rope you can find; this will help build your grip. If you can't find a rope of at least an inch in diameter or more, purchase two thinner ropes about three feet long and tape the two ropes together, making one thick rope.

Now that your rope is ready, all you have to do is loop your rope over the chin-up bar at your local gym. If you don't train at a gym or don't have a chin-up bar at home, you will need to find a sturdy tree branch or beam to loop the rope over. Once you loop the rope over your bar, you will grab each end of the rope with each hand. You can now do chin-ups hanging from the rope. You will have to really grip tightly to keep your grip from sliding off the ends of the rope. This will give you the same benefits as rope climbing. If you can't do chin-ups in this style, just hang from the rope as long as you can. You can develop tremendous lower arm strength from this exercise as well as upper arm and upper back strength. As you get stronger, you can tie a little weight around your waist to keep improving. This exercise is profitable to all, but if you are a heavier athlete, this is your way to achieve your grip strength goals.

Finger Walking

The exercise that I call finger walking is a special exercise that I ran across several years ago. I stumbled across it while playing around with a sledgehammer in my back yard. Finger walking is easily one of the

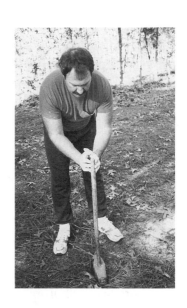

John positions his fingers on the tip of the sledgehammer handle (left), and begins to walk them down the handle (below left) until he reaches the bottom (below right). John gives this movement top marks, as a way to both strengthen the fingers and increase their dexterity. Photos by Steve Jeck.

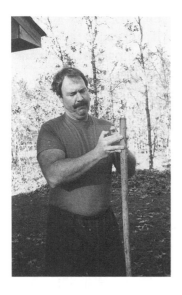

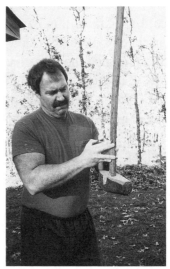

best ways I have found to develop finger strength. It will equally develop each finger, for it works all the fingers to their utmost. This exercise is also a great way to develop tremendous dexterity. It is great for the piano player, as well as the rock climber.

All that is needed is a sledgehammer and some patience. Most men can't finger walk with an 8-lb. sledgehammer, so you may want to start out with a 6-lb. hammer as you can always add weight to the hammer. Once you get a feel for this exercise, it will become very enjoyable.

To start, lift your hammer straight in front of you, with the head of the hammer toward the ground and the handle of the hammer facing upward (follow photos closely.) You should have the fingertips of each hand on the outsides of the handle. In other words, your hands should be as if you're clapping them with the handle of the hammer between your hands at the tips of your fingers. Once you're holding the hammer off the ground with the handle between your fingertips, start to move or walk your fingers down the shaft of the hammer. This will start to move the whole hammer upward little by little. You will start with your fingers at the top of the hammer handle and end up at the head of the hammer. This will feel awkward at first; however, if you are patient and follow the photos closely, you will soon have a feel for this great finger strength developer. Be sure to keep your hands and fingers straight as if you were clapping, and also be sure to use just your fingertips to move the hammer handle upward.

You can do this exercise over and over for endurance, or you can go heavy and complete the finger walking one set at a time. As you get stronger, you can slide a 2-1/2 or five-lb. weight plate down the shaft of the hammer to make it heavier. If you don't have weights, you can use duct tape to tape a brick to the bottom of the head of the hammer. Try finger walking for a while and you will make great gains in your grip.

Chapter Five

Training with Block Weights

As a professional strongman, I am often asked which one exercise or device do I think is the best for developing a strong grip. First of all, that is a very hard question. There are so many ways to train the lower arms. Also some methods are better than others for different sports or different feats of strength. A powerlifter who wants to be able to hold onto that big deadlift might need a different routine than a rock climber, or a martial artist may require a different style of exercise than a gymnast.

While all exercises for the lower arms have their place, some are simply better than others. For the past two years I have been training very hard with different block weights. These block weights are mostly the heads of dumbbells I have cut off. These weights are different shapes and sizes: Some are hexagon-shaped and some are more rounded shapes. I have been doing different exercises and playing different games with these weights, and I have noticed that I have gained more strength in my hands and fingers than with any other type of training. I have also enjoyed these block weights more than any other training that I have ever done before. This of course means more motivation, resulting in bigger gains. Also, the dexterity of all the fingers is brought into play, resulting in better muscle control.

Once again these block weights vary in size and thickness. These different thicknesses result in the use of your hands at different angles.

For example, with a 25-lb. block weight, your hand may be opened about halfway, but with a 45-lb. block weight your hand will be opened much wider. These varying widths of your hands grasping the weights will work your grip in many different ways.

Many people have strength with their hands in a certain position or when their hand is opened a certain width, but this type of block weight training will allow and enable the trainee to develop a pinch grip strength at every width that their hand will open. This type of strength will be very useful in all sports as well as in any type of test of strength. Another huge advantage block weights have over other types of grip training is that the thumb is constantly being used. Many strength athletes have a powerful grasp when it comes to gripping a bar for deadlifting or squeezing a heavy-duty handgripper closed, but when it comes to any type of pinch gripping they do poorly because of an under-developed thumb.

The martial artist who is involved in any style where the hand is used to claw or gouge will really benefit from a good block weight program. Also, the explosiveness required for clawing-type strikes will be developed by tossing block weights from hand to hand, not to mention the eye-hand coordination.

A rock climber who needs fingertip strength and muscle control will also benefit from the block weights because the holds on the block weights would simulate some of the hand holds on the rocks. Also the individual finger grips on the block weights would help where added finger strength on the rocks is needed.

We just briefly discussed two sports that would benefit. The use of block weights is, in my opinion, the best way to develop strength of hand and forearm, from the top of the forearms to the tips of the fingers. You can also make tremendous gains in thumb strength from handling block weights. They are truly a great way to gain lower arm strength that can be used for any task, and a lot of fun can be had with them.

I do a lot of prison ministry where I speak from the Word of God. I also do feats of strength to get the inmates' respect and attention. I always take several block weights of different sizes to challenge them to lift in different ways. These weights seem to steal the show. They always get a big laugh and everyone wants to try and lift them. I often take smaller block weights that they can lift. I also take larger blocks and do feats of strength that I haven't seen duplicated. It can be amusing to watch people trying to lift heavy block weights off the floor. The weights seem to be literally glued to the floor. Lifting a heavy block weight off the ground in a one-hand pinch grip has to be the most deceptive test of strength I've ever seen.

I like to use the York dumbbell heads, for they are a kind of roundish shape, making them more difficult to lift. You may find many different weights to use for these exercises, but we will examine the York and Ivanko weights, for they are probably the best to use and they are also easy to acquire.

Let's start with the York weights first. Go out and find a sporting goods shop or a business that specializes in gym equipment. Find a York dumbbell that weighs between 45 and 60 pounds. This is a weight that I would suggest starting with; even if you have strong hands, this weight will give you a very good workout. After you buy your dumbbell, you will need to cut the ends off, leaving you with the two block weights.* I know you are probably saying, "This is a lot of money, and now he wants me to cut off the ends." Remember two things I'm telling you: 1) this is a way that will surely help your hand strength jump up drastically, and 2) these block weights will last forever.

Now that you have two weights around 25 to 30 pounds, you are ready to begin. Oh, in case you're wondering how a weight from 25 to 30 pounds is going to help when you have heard of guys pinch gripping over 100 pounds with one hand, consider the following. First, if you're looking at the York block in front of you, you have probably already noticed that it is wider than plates. This of course opens your hand wider, making it more difficult to lift. But what makes it even harder is the shape of the York block, which fans outward, making it wider at the middle of the weight than at the top. This spreads out your hand even more. With a regular pinch grip on weightlifting plates or on a home-made pinch block, your hand goes straight down over the weight, completely vertical. This makes it much easier than if the weight flares outward like your York block weight. This wider grip makes it harder.

For your information, I have found that a person can pinch grip about twice the weight on a regular pinch grip then you can on this flaring style of block weight. Just about everyone I've seen seems to fall into this range. Another factor is hand size; some people who have smaller hands are unable to get a good grip on a heavy block weight. Most block weights get wider as they get heavier, including our York weights. The 50-lb. weight from a York 100-lb. dumbbell is very wide.

*Editor's Note: See Appendix 1: How to Make Your Own Thick-Handled Dumbbells, for more details on how to do this.

My hands are a little smaller than average and I can just barely get a grip on this 50-lb. block weight.

This gives the smaller-handed man a disadvantage on the bigger weights; however, through work I have been able to lift the biggest of block weights. For safety, always remember not to grip too wide or where your hand has to reach out too far. This can cause your thumb to hyperextend. If you injure your thumb, it will be slow to heal. Remember, start with smaller block weights and work your way up. Once you get used to this type of grip training you will be able to grip with your hand opened wider. Let your thumb get used to the load it's supporting.

To give you an idea of what a good lift is with a York block weight, I'll tell you this. You may search the world over and never find a man who can lift the York 50-lb. block. It is so wide and has such an outward flare, it is a tremendous challenge to any grip man. Richard Sorin has had a York 50-lb. block in his gym for a long time and countless strength athletes have tried to lift it without success. No one that Richard has seen has even broken it off the ground an inch except Richard. As you may know, Richard Sorin was the first man to close the IronMind #3 gripper. As tough as closing the #3 is, Richard feels that pinch gripping this 50-lb. York block weight is even harder. Just recently I got a 50-lb. York block out and found that I am now able to lift it in a one-handed pinch grip, which shows you how much the handling of block weights has improved my grip.*

I have also noticed that a 30-lb. York block weight is about the size that stops most people. If you have a strong grip and train your hands a lot, you will probably be able to lift this weight. However, if your grip isn't very good this may get the best of you. I have seen some pretty strong weight-trained men not be able to lift this 30-lb. block. For most people with fairly strong hands the 25-lb. block weights will be perfect for training. We will now look at some exercises with your block weights. There are many movements and challenging games you can use to develop those hands. I will not try to put the whole course of exercises in this book. However, I will put a handful of what I think to be some of the better ones to start you on the road to grip success.

Editor's Note: As we go to press, John has lifted this "block" with an additional five pounds attached to it—a feat no one else in the world has performed.

Exercise 1: Block Toss

For this exercise you will need just one block. You may also want to use a little bit of chalk on the block and also on your hands. I often do these exercises outside, but if you live in the city and don't have a back yard, you can use a piece of plywood on the floor to place your blocks on. This plywood will also absorb the shock from a block that slips from your grasp. Special note: Nicely explain this and your wife or

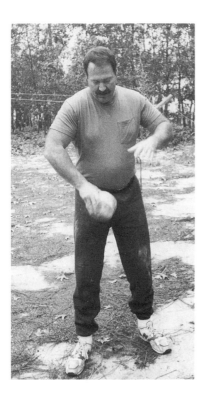

John tosses a block from hand to hand, a top movement for boosting thumb strength. Photo by Steve Jeck.

mother will surely understand and let you play with your blocks in your house or apartment.

Tossing block weights from hand to hand is one of the best exercises for the grip that could ever be done. First, grasp a smaller block weight. Always grip the weight with your hand over the top, as in a traditional pinch grip. This will constantly work the grip. Start lifting your weight with one hand; now toss it in front of you and grab it with the other hand. Once again, when catching it, always grab it with your hand directly over the top. Some people want to have their wrist turned so that the pressure is on the biceps and wrist instead of the grip.

Just toss it from hand to hand until your hands tire; you may not be able to catch it at first. If that's the case, just pass it from hand to hand. This will give you the same effect. As you improve, try to catch it with two fingers instead of the whole hand. If you are unable to lift it with both hands, just practice deadlifting it. This will develop the strength for you to toss the blocks in the future.

This block tossing exercise will really build hand strength as well as develop an explosive grip. This exercise is perfect for the martial artist who is trying to build strength for clawing techniques, as well as gain eye-hand coordination.

Exercise 2: Farmer's Walk

The second exercise is the farmer's walk. This is a very challenging exercise. Simply pinch grip the blocks one in each hand and carry them as far as you can. You may have a weaker hand and have to drop one weight before the other. This exercise will help develop both hands equally. You can also carry one block weight at a time and pick a certain distance to walk. As the hand carrying the weight tires, change it to the other hand and continue walking. If you live in the city and can't get out to perform this exercise, you can hold the block weights as long as you can. I often carry a block weight down the street tossing it from hand to hand as I walk. Always remember in this exercise or in any exercise using the block weights, never hold them against your body. This would be lightening the load and defeating the purpose.

Exercise 3: Clean and Press

The next exercise is the clean and press. This can be performed with a weight in each hand or with one hand at a time. I would suggest doing this one with a weight in each hand. This is a very difficult exercise and also a very important one. Unless you have a very strong grip, you will have to perform this exercise with a block weight of around 25 pounds.

Start by deadlifting the weights off the ground. Now, while holding the weights in a deadlift position, lift them up to your shoulders, cleaning them. The clean to your shoulders can be done with a quick burst or with a slow steady movement. Now with the blocks at your shoulders, press them overhead, then lower them back to the shoulders and then down to the standing deadlift position again. Now repeat the entire

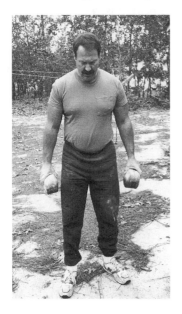 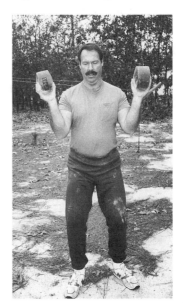

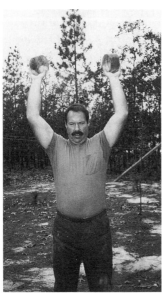

John demonstrates the clean and press while pinch gripping a pair of his block weights. Photos by Steve Jeck.

movement again and again. Do as many repetitions as you can. You will find out that this is a difficult exercise and that it is also a key exercise in the program. You will also notice that after the press overhead, when you are lowering the weight back to the deadlift position, the weight feels much heavier. This, of course, is gravity working against your grip, and in this case gravity is our friend.

If you can only do this exercise for one rep, just keep repeating the movement as you can. If you decide to do this exercise one hand at a time, always remember to do equal sets with both hands. As you improve you can use heavier block weights. You can also do this clean and press exercise or any of these movements with fewer fingers on the block. Using fewer fingers develops strength as well as muscle control.

Exercise 4: Snatch Lift

Another great exercise with block weights is the snatch lift. This may be a little hard at first, for it demands a very good grip. All of these movements once developed can be used as feats of strength. So if some of them seem hard at first, hang in there. To perform the snatch lift I would start using just one block weight at first.

Standing over the weight, grasp the weight in a pinch grip, and all at once pull and lift the weight overhead in one continuous movement. From there, ease the block weight down to the ground and repeat the movement. This lift is very hard with a York block weight of 40 pounds. I have been lifting this weight in the snatch lift for a while now, but I have not seen anyone else be able to duplicate it. I have seen many powerful men with great grips fall way short on this lift with 40 pounds.

From, what I've seen, I would say that a snatch with a 25-lb. block weight is fairly good, so if you can't perform this with a 25-lb. weight, don't feel bad. If you continue to train with block weights, you will soon be performing this feat.

Exercise 5: Individual Finger lifts

Earlier, I mentioned lifting the block weights with individual fingers as you improve. As your weights get easier, you should start lifting the blocks with just the index and middle fingers on one side and, of course, your thumb on the other side. You still want to use your whole hand for most of the harder lifts, but the fewer number of fingers on the block will really strengthen them.

If you can get to where you can lift a 25-lb. York block in each hand using only the index finger and thumb, you will be reaching a very high level. One step further would be lifting them in this manner and then cleaning and pressing them. Also, what may be even harder is tossing them hand to hand, catching them with one finger. These methods will really develop great finger strength as well as dexterity and muscle control.

Exercise 6: Follow the Leader

I will mention one more method of grip training that is fun and useful with blocks. I call it follow the leader. If you have a grip partner, hand him a block weight. Now as you pick up your weight, he has to pick up his. Whatever you do, he has to also do. There are countless maneuvers to do with the blocks. You can, of course, clean and press the block, toss it from hand to hand, or simply just hold it. To get a little fancier, you can change hands behind your back and also change hands between your legs. This game will push your grip to the utmost. If you do not have a partner to practice with, follow the leader is just as useful going through these maneuvers by yourself.

As far as endurance goes, I will mention a feat that you may want to shoot for down the road. With a 25-lb. York block weight, I was able to toss it from hand to hand for 25 minutes. As you might guess, my lower arms were pretty tired.

These exercises will be more than enough to get you started. You may find different exercises and games to play with your blocks. I mentioned earlier that York dumbbells were the best weights to use for cutting off the bar and making your own block weights. I also have some Ivanko blocks. These blocks off the Ivankos are not as wide as the Yorks. They also do not flare out as far as the Yorks. This, of course, allows you to lift more. I think the Yorks are the best, but if you want to use Ivankos, they are good as well. You should be able to find these weights, but if you can't, you can find a York dealer by calling the York Barbell Company in York, Pennsylvania.

Some of you may be wondering, "How about using a large dumbbell without cutting off the ends and just grasping a block with each hand and deadlifting?" Good question. First you will find that this will put your wrist in a slight bind, which in time may develop not only pain, but injuries. Second, it is very important to have individual weights to do the exercises. You will not be able to toss them from hand to hand with the bar in the middle, which is the foundation of grip development on block weights. Your thumb will also be put in great stress. We won't go on from here—just cut off the bar. You will be more than pleased.

I guess by now you know I think a lot of block weight training. As far as block weights go, I will leave you with this: *Block Weight Training = Grip Strength.*

Chapter Six

Training with Thick-Handled Dumbbells

Thick-handled dumbbells have always been a favorite of the professional strongmen of old, whether it be for a challenge lift or simply for training. They are truly one of the best ways to develop lower arm strength. If you ever find any pictures of old training equipment, or if you ever go to the York Museum in Pennsylvania, you will notice that most of the old dumbbells have thick handles. This was simply the rule of thumb in those days. As the times changed, the handles all became the regular size that you see and use now. Also in past times lifters were more concerned about their performance. Now in these modern times many people who lift weights are lifting so they can build up simply to look good.*

Our goal of grip strength does not come into use on the posing platform, so grip strength has been forgotten by most modern bodybuilders. Grip strength also cannot be detected by merely looking at someone, so here again it has no use for those who are training to walk around on the beach.

*Editor's Note: Grip aside, a lot of old-time dumbbells had to have thick handles—the materials of the day were too weak to make thinner handles strong enough for the task.

First, let's address the problem of the thickness. You will not want a handle less than two inches in diameter, as this would be defeating the purpose. You will also not want a handle over three inches in diameter unless you have a gigantic hand—not a big hand, but gigantic. If you use a shaft that is way too big, it can put excessive stress on the thumb. So we are shooting for something from two inches to three inches in diameter. An important note to remember is that most of the famous strongmen of the past used dumbbells with a handle around 2-1/2 inches thick. This is also my advice to you. If you have small hands, a two-inch shaft may be best; if you have exceptionally large hands, a three-inch shaft will be all right. For a person with normal-sized hands, let's stick to 2-1/2 inches.

Now our next question is how heavy a dumbbell should be used. Most of you will be using your dumbbell for training your grip, not for a challenge lift. For training you will have to remember that a dumbbell with a thick handle feels much heavier than a dumbbell with a normal handle. Remember when we talked about the strongmen of old, we spoke of the famous Thomas Inch dumbbell that was about 2-1/2 inches thick at the handle and weighed 172 lbs. Remember also there were only a handful of men throughout time that could deadlift this dumbbell. Using this as a gauge, we learn that our weight for training is going to be cut way down. Dennis Rogers had a dumbbell with a 2-3/8 inch handle and weighing 126 lbs. that he let people try to lift for fun. He did this, trying to find out just how hard a feat this was to lift. Many people tried and only a couple of people succeeded. Also, all of these people were men who trained with weights.

I would say that a man with a good grip would probably want to train with a dumbbell of about 50 to 70 lbs. on a 2-1/2 inch handle. This training would consist of exercises like one-arm rows, shrugs, curls, and cleans. A very strong man with a great grip could probably train with more. If you haven't used weights much or you don't have very strong hands, I would start with a weight of around 30 lbs. I have explained how you can make your own thick-handled dumbbell bars in Appendix 1.

A great exercise for the grip done with a thick-handled dumbbell is simply carrying it or holding it as long as you can. Once you get a feel for the dumbbell, it's great for tossing from hand to hand. I actually find this the best training with a thick-handled dumbbell. This will develop an explosive grip that will help in all sports. This tossing action will also help develop both hands equally.

You may wonder how to progress as the weight becomes easier to handle. Of course you can do more repetitions or carry the dumbbell for longer distances. This will, of course, develop more endurance, which is important, but if you want to gain more raw strength in your lower arms, other measures are required. You will, however, want to use the original weight for a while to gain the strength you need to progress to tougher dumbbells, especially if you aren't used to training your grip in this manner.

As you progress I would strongly suggest that you invest in a heavier thick-handled dumbbell. In the long run you can't go wrong with such an investment. However, if you don't or can't invest more money in another dumbbell, there are other alternatives.*

You may want to simply make the handle thicker by adding tape to the shaft. Remember in the modern day profiles in Chapter 1. how John Ottarski uses the same weight, but adds a strand of tape to the handle with every workout. This will give you the same results in your grip strength improvement as if you added more weight. If you are dead set on adding more weight to the dumbbell and don't want to have another one made, you can have a welder weld a small weight plate to either the sides of the dumbbell or possibly underneath the bottom of the dumb-bell. This may not look pretty, but the results will still be the same. You may also take a couple of small weight discs and tape them to each side of the weight. In the grip game you must be innovative.

You can't go wrong with thick-handled dumbbells. This is a big reason why the old-timers had such powerful hands and such sinewy forearms.

Training with Kettlebells

It is amazing how many telephone calls and letters I receive from people wanting to find kettlebells. First of all, they are very hard to find and second, finding someone who will sell you their antique kettlebells is about as hard as becoming the king of France.

I have explained in detail two ways you can make kettlebells which have the same traditional use as the originals (see Appendix 2.). Once again since this is a book on grip strength, I would suggest you use thick

---

*Editor's Note: One-piece dumbbells certainly have their appeal, but now you can see the big advantages of plate-loading dumbbells—the weight can be adjusted as required.

handles. I have made a collection of kettlebells over the last couple of years and they are a very good tool for the development of lower arm strength as well as overall upper body strength. They were very popular in the Eastern bloc countries and still are used in certain areas. The Soviets liked to train with kettlebells to gain hand strength. A favorite exercise was forming a circle and tossing the kettlebells from one person to another. This, of course, forced the catcher to catch the kettlebell by the handle, bringing into play the muscles of the hand and fingers. If you don't have a group or even a partner, you can just toss the kettlebell from hand to hand.

Several years ago I saw three Mongolian strongmen in a circus who had some very heavy-looking kettlebells. The weight of the kettlebells was not mentioned, but they looked to be in the neighborhood of 80 to 100 lbs. The three strongmen stood in a small circle and tossed the kettlebells to one another with great skill. They appeared to catch the kettlebells with just their fingertips. When they finished they threw the kettlebells into the air, letting them crash to the floor with a loud bang. By doing this exercise with heavy kettlebells, the strongmen had developed very strong fingers. The handles on their kettlebells appeared to be of normal size. The handles on my kettlebells are almost three inches in diameter. This puts much more pressure on the hands, which is our goal.

Kettlebell swings are a tremendous all-around exercise that really works the grip. If you want to make them into an even better grip exercise, try alternating hands in midair. For example, if you are doing a kettlebell swing with your right hand, let go of the kettlebell at about shoulder height and immediately grasp it with your left hand. Continue down, start the next swing with your left hand, let go of the kettlebell at about shoulder height, and grasp it with your right hand. Repeat this movement, alternating hands in each swing.

Chapter Seven

More Training for the Lower Arms and Fingers

Let's look at a few well-known exercises that are used to develop the lower arms.

Wrist Curls

First let's look at the wrist curl. What a classic forearm builder. I have done them myself for years and years. Many trainers tell athletes to "do a few sets of these and you will develop a great grip." As we talked about earlier, I feel that forearm size and grip strength are two different things. It's like calling an English man a Scottish man. Just because they are from the same region does not mean they are the same. Wrist curls are a good lower arm exercise, and they should be included in your routine. They will help pump your forearm and strengthen your wrist, which is a must, and they will also help add flexibility to your wrists. However, if you are waiting for them to build your hand strength to new heights, you will be waiting with the same person who is waiting to win a million dollars in the lottery. I would suggest doing standard wrist curls (palms up) as well as reverse wrist curls (palms down) in your training routine. I would use them first as a wrist builder, and second as a warm-up for more isolated training for your hands.

Curling Weight Plates

In my opinion, this book would not be complete if this tremendous wrist and finger exercise were left out. Curling regular weight plates may be the greatest wrist developer under the sun. You might ask "if it is so great, then why haven't I ever heard of it?" Well, that is a good question. The fact is that you may not even know anyone who has ever heard of it. To the best of my knowledge, it has never been mentioned in a training book past or present. There were a handful of strongmen from years ago who performed this exercise to help develop their extraordinary lower arm strength.

All you need are basic weight disks found at any gym. You simply grasp a plate in a pinch grip position. In other words, stand the plate vertically on the floor and grip it with your hand over the top. Your four fingers will be on one side of the plate and your thumb on the other side. Now grip tightly and deadlift the plate. Once in this position, curl the plate to your chest in the same fashion you would perform any type of curl. Now lower the plate back to the deadlift position, then curl again and again. It will save time if you use a plate in each hand and curl the plates in alternate fashion.

You will quickly notice that a great deal of stress is placed on the wrist. Try to keep your wrist stable and straight throughout the whole movement. If your wrist is being bent back, you are using too much weight. This exercise is so difficult because much of the weight is away from the hand.

As far as picking the right plate, remember that the heavier the weight, the harder, and the longer the plate, the harder it becomes as well, for the leverage against you becomes greater. If your wrists are pretty strong, you can probably use a 25-lb. plate. If your wrists are not strong, you can sandwich two 10-lb. plates together using a pinch grip. If this is too much, use one 10-lb. plate. If you can perform reps with 35-lb. plates, you have very strong wrists. If you can curl a 45-lb. or 50-lb. plate with one hand, consider yourself having some of the strongest wrists in the world. Curling a 45-lb. or 50-lb. plate is included in the chapter on challenge exercises (Chapter 11, Testing Your Endurance: Can You Muster This?).

A very important note to remember is that while curling plates is a great exercise to build wrist strength beyond your wildest dreams, great stress is placed on the wrist as well. Do not use plates that are too heavy and never attempt to plate curl beyond your strength—you may strain your wrists. Well, good luck and good plate curling.

Sand Grabbing

Another popular grip training method is sand grabbing. This is simply thrusting your hand into a bucket of sand. There are basically two methods. One is grabbing the sand as quickly and explosively as possible. The other is jamming your hand as far into the sand as possible with your fingers completely straight. These two methods were developed in ancient China for kung fu practitioners to develop strength for their clawing and striking techniques. These methods are productive for developing a strong explosive grip. However, it is very important to be very explosive with the training. You must give it your all if you are going to improve.

Sand grabbing also has its own method of improvement. As the sand becomes easier to thrust into, you can load the bucket with harder substances. The ultimate in training is being able to thrust your hand deep into steel shot. Do not go out and try to jam your fingers into steel shot—you may badly injure your fingers. If you like the sound of this type of training, start with the sand and get a feel for it before you try to move to a harder substance. If you are patient and put the effort into sand grabbing, you will get a hand up on the others.

Lever Lifts or Weaver Sticks

Another classic way to develop a strong grip and a great pair of forearms is the traditional lever lifting or Weaver stick. These lifts have been and can be done in many different ways. However, we will look at the simplest method. Just take an axe, shovel, or even a pitch fork and lay it on the ground. Now grab the end of the handle and lift the tool off the ground. You have to lock your wrist to keep the end of the tool from hitting the ground. If your wrist isn't strong enough, the weighted end of the tool won't clear the ground. It is important to use only your wrist to lever up the weight.

As you improve, you can use sledgehammers to lever up. Few men can lever up a 10-lb. sledgehammer. If you have a sledgehammer and can't lever it up by the end of the handle, lift it as far down the shaft as you can. Lever lifting is a great exercise for wrist development. It is used by professional arm wrestlers quite often. It is an excellent exercise for baseball players as well.

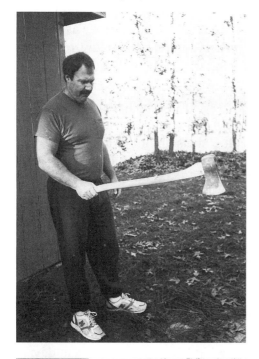

John levers an axe to the front...

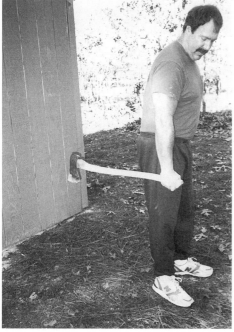

...and to the back. Photos by Steve Jeck.

Wrist Rollers

The final exercise we will look at is the wrist roller. This is an exercise where a weight is added to a rope or chain and then attached to a short stick or bar. The weight dangles at the end of the rope while the trainee rolls the rope around the stick, using his wrists. This was a favorite exercise of the great John Grimek. John's forearms were some of the greatest forearms of all time, by the way. The wrist roller is a great lower arm developer. You don't see it used much today. When you use the wrist roller you should roll it up and then down without any rest. This will develop both parts of your forearm.

To make the exercise more difficult and also more productive, use a stick or bar with a thick handle. Two inches in diameter would be a good handle for this exercise. An interesting training method for wrist rolling is to add a few strands of tape around the shaft with every work-out, making the handle thicker little by little. The results will be thicker forearms and a stronger grip.

John Ottarski's Baseball Lift

Just recently I was introduced to a new exercise for building the grip. John Ottarski of Durham, North Carolina, told me about an exercise he started doing. John, of course, is profiled in Chapter 1. on present day gripmasters. He is a tremendous grip strength practitioner. He excels in all types of lower arm strength. John took an ordinary baseball, drilled a hole through the middle, and then hammered a 60-penny nail through the hole. Once the nail was through the baseball he bent the end of the nail double, forming a hook. Once this was completed, he was able to attach weights onto the baseball by attaching a chain or threading a small rope through the hook. Now John gripped the baseball with his hand over the top of the ball and lifted. Instantly he realized that this was a world-class way of developing a great grip.

After I was introduced to this exercise, I went out and bought a baseball as well as a softball. I made this grip blaster out of both the baseball and the softball. I found that I prefer the softball over the baseball because it is bigger and harder to grasp. I would strongly suggest that you make this gadget yourself. It is absolutely one of the best trainers I have ever found. The choice is yours; you can make either the baseball or the softball. I myself use both to train with. You can do deadlifts or one-handed rows, or just hold the weight as long as you can.

Lifting the ball with your hand over the top is like an eagle with its talons grasping its prey. Do not cup your hand under the ball. Be sure to grasp the ball over the top for the best results.

When making your ball, be sure to drill a hole through the middle of the ball that is slightly smaller than the nail. For instance, drill a 3/16 inch hole through the ball and then drive your 1/4 inch thick 60-penny nail through the hole. You will now want to place your ball in a vise to steady the ball. Place a pair of pliers at the end of the nail. You will probably want to place another piece of steel up against the nail where it is coming through the ball. This will act as a brace as you bend the end of the nail into a hook with the pliers. After the nail is bent toward the ball, take a hammer to finish knocking the end of the nail against the ball, forming the hook. You are now ready to put a chain or rope through the hook and start lifting. One note: If you decide to make the softball, you may want to use a longer nail than the 60-penny nail. A seven-inch nail would be better if you can find one. If you can't find a longer nail than the 60-penny, go ahead and use the 60-penny. However, you may want to place your chain or rope against the ball when you bend the end into a hook. This will ensure that you can get your rope or chain through the hook.

This exercise will work your entire hand. I have found that lifting these balls is a great way to develop tremendous thumb strength.

Fingertip Push-ups

Fingertip push-ups have been used for years and years to develop finger strength. They are a favorite of martial artists and rock climbers. One reason, I think, has made them a favorite, and that is they require no equipment and they can also be done anywhere and anytime. They also have their own system for improvement. For instance, as your fingers get stronger, you can do the push-ups on three, two, or even one finger. You can occasionally even find someone doing push-ups on his thumbs. I think myself that fingertip push-ups are a good way to develop finger strength for certain activities. A rock climber, for instance, can benefit from such a program. On the other hand, if you're trying to develop a strong crushing grip, I would look elsewhere.

One more very important point to be made is that like rope climbing, fingertip push-up trainees are usually light in bodyweight. This, of course, does not put the pressure on their fingers like that of a heavier trainee. Overall, I think that fingertip push-ups are good way to cross-train in a routine. A heavy person can profit from them in particular.

Finger Extension—Jar Lifting

A very important point that needs to be made is that we always think of closing the hand when we think of grip strength. We never think of the muscles that open the hand. I have found in the last couple of years that by adding a movement which works the muscles that open the hand, my overall grip strength has improved. These types of exercises are never included in hand strength routines. Actually I have found quite a few exercises that work these muscles. We will touch on a few.

One exercise I like to perform is with a large jar like a cookie jar or even a mason jar. I fill the jar with steel shot and put my fingers inside the very top of the jar. From here I lift the jar using only the pressure from my fingers inside the top of the jar. When you first try this exercise you will probably not have much strength using your hand in this position. As you train, you will increase your strength fairly rapidly with this movement. These muscles are potentially stronger than you think they are. When you start lifting these jars in this manner you can use steel shot, sand, or even water to fill the jars. I like to use a weight that I can hold for about 30 seconds. You can also lift the jars with three, two, or even one finger to make it more difficult. Be careful not to cut yourself on the edge of the jar. You may want to use a little tape around the lip of the jar.

Finger Extension—Sand Bucket

Another way to train the muscles that open your hand is to use a bucket of sand. Put your hand into the sand and make a fist. With your hand in a fist, open your hand, forcibly resisting against the sand. Repeat this over and over, using both hands equally. I feel that a program of high repetitions is the most productive with the sand. I like to do one set with each hand and repeat until exhausted. Once you start to include exercises opening your hand, you will feel a new strength in your fingers.

Finger Extension Bands

One last way we will look at is to open your hand using bands or surgical tubing. Simply wrap the bands or tubing around your hand and open your fingers against the resistance of the bands. I would suggest using high repetitions on this exercise as well.

Add an exercise using the muscles it takes to open your hand and your grip will climb to new heights.

Chapter Eight

Manual Labor and Thick-Handled Tools

I want to mention a subject that may surprise you. That subject is manual labor. Many times you will find men with strong grips and powerful forearms that have not ever lifted a weight in their lives. This is because they have worked hard with their hands on their daily jobs.

The hand dynamometer, a device used to measure gripping force, has shown that the average man can squeeze about 112 pounds of pressure with his right hand. This number is not very high. Most men from years ago, whether athletic or not, would have been able to squeeze a higher number for the simple fact that they used their hands on the job or on the farm. At times I like to take heavy-duty grippers around with me for people to try. I've found that men who do manual labor usually test higher on these grippers than men who just train with weights.

For the last seven years or so I have done a lot of manual labor as well as special grip training—anywhere from using an axe to using a pick and shovel. This work has really helped me with my lower arm training. It will hit muscles that weights never can.

If you look at the competitors in the lumberjack events—you know, the events where they chop through logs for time and where they use a crosscut saw for time—these men all have strong powerful hands from this great stress that's put on them. Most of them don't even know what a bench press or a barbell curl is. However, there are not many body-builders who would want to compete with them in feats of hand and wrist strength.

Another popular work chore that was also used as a test of strength is the manly art of wheelbarrow pushing. Anyone who has worked laying brick or stone knows what it's like to push a heavy wheelbarrow loaded with mortar or concrete through a muddy construction site. If you've pushed many, you probably know what it's like to turn one over as well. A viselike grip is required for this chore, and to keep your wheelbarrow upright.

In Canada it has been a longtime test of strength to push heavy wheelbarrows for distance and also at times uphill—only these wheel-barrows are specially made, able to hold thousands of pounds. One must lift these wheelbarrows in a partial deadlift-type maneuver and then walk as far as he can.

I have spoken to a couple of old-time competitors as well as some present day champs and they all said that the grip is the key element. I used to push a regular working-type wheelbarrow up and down a hill for a half-hour straight to train for stamina. As I look back on this workout, my grip was the last thing I was concerned about, yet it was my hands that were the most fatigued at the end of the thirty minutes.

Let's also look at the men who used to drive the spikes on the rail-road with a 16-lb. hammer. Times have changed and I understand this is not done very often any more, but just think of doing this all day. What a workout. Or, what about Slim "The Hammerman" Farman from Pottstown, Pennsylvania. Slim is one of the best strongmen of all time. He is now in his sixties and still performing. He is the undisputed champion of levering heavy sledgehammers. This is a test of strength practiced by laborers as well as a feat seen on stage with professional strongmen. In these feats, the hammers are lifted off the ground by grasping the ends of the handle, and they are also tilted by the ends of the handle so that the head of hammer touches the nose or the forehead of the performer. Slim has taken this feat to a level all his own. Slim is a professional stonecutter by trade—a trade that finds him breaking stones with a 16-lb. sledgehammer all day. This difficult job has cer-tainly developed a foundation of strength that helps Slim on the stage.

Let's look at one more craft that demands as well as develops a powerful set of lower arms. The iceman of the cities was the man who was always a popular character. He had the difficult job of delivering blocks of ice. He would find a parking place as close as he could and grab his ice tongs and a block of ice, and he was off. Ice came in blocks of 50 and 100 pounds, so it was no easy task, considering he had to carry these blocks of ice up flights of stairs and often a hundred yards down the street. Let's also remember there was no time to stop and rest when you had someone's ice out in the sun.

I've read and heard about Joseph Mongelli, an iceman from New York City, who in the early 1900s used to carry these heavy blocks of ice for blocks before he would set them down, or carry block after block of ice up flights of stairs. He had developed world class strength in his hands and wrists. Or what about August Johnson, an iceman who at age 64 carried a 32-lb. bag of coins with one hand without letting the bag touch his body for a distance of one mile before setting the bag down. An incredible feat.

With all of today's comforts, we have gotten away from using our hands outside of gym workouts or outside of squeezing grippers, but don't forget the way farmers and laborers of the past developed their strong hands. Also, your hands and wrists can't determine the difference between a barbell and an axe.

Chapter Nine

Goals and Training Programs

The secret to success at any goal is to stay motivated. This is not always as easy as it sounds. Oftentimes goals seem so far away that we lose our motivation. I have found that working on small goals keeps me more motivated. Also, by achieving small goals one after the other makes life very challenging in a fun way.

With our goal of developing tremendous gripping power, this system of motivation holds true as well. Grip strength, unlike some other types of strength, is not always quick to develop. We are dealing with tendons and smaller muscle groups that do not always respond as quickly as we would like. This is one reason I have a lot of what appear to be strange, offbeat exercises in this book. To develop a special kind of grip strength, you need special kinds of grip exercises.

If you stick with these exercises, you will consistently improve. Make them fun by setting small goals to accomplish. Be sure to include the different kinds of grip strength in your routines. For instance, include an exercise for crushing strength, an exercise for pinch gripping power which will also develop your thumbs, and also include an exercise which works the muscles which open your hand. Change different exercises around if you get bored with or tired of one. Little by little strive to improve on each exercise. If you stay loyal to your training and keep your sight on your goal, you will achieve grip strength greatness.

Table A.
Do These Exercises to Develop These Areas of Grip and Lower Arm Strength

Exercises	Indiv. fingers	Hand—pinching, thumb	Hand—vise grip, crushing	Wrist	Forearm	Lower arm general	Upper body	Explosive grip
• Thick-handled DB's			X		X	X	X	
• Kettlebells	X		X		X	X	X	
• Block Weights	X	X			X	X		
- Block Toss	X	X						
- Farmer's Walk		X				X		
- Clean & Press		X					X	
- Snatch Lift		X					X	
- Indiv. Finger	X	X						
- Follow the Leader		X				X		
• Telegraph Key	X							
• Heavy-duty Handgrippers			X		X	X		
• Wire Cutting			X		X	X		
• Plier Lifting			X					
• Double Hammer Squeeze			X					
• Grip Machine			X		X			
• Bag Catching			X					X
• Anvil Lifting (horn)			X					
• Anvil Lifting (pinch)		X						
• Wide Timber Lifting		X						
• Weight Plate Lifting		X						
• Board Lifting		X						
• Mr. Pinch-O-Grip		X						
• Axe Head Lifting		X						
• Rope Climbing			X	X	X	X	X	
• Finger Walking	X							
• Wrist Curls				X	X			
• Curling Weight Plates	X			X	X	X		
• Fingertip Push-ups	X							
• Sand Grabbing	X			X	X	X		X
• Lever Lift/Weaver Stick				X	X			
• Wrist Roller				X	X	X		
• Baseball Lift		X				X		
• Finger Extension	X							
• Pulling Cut Nails	X	X						
• Nail Bending			X	X	X	X	X	
• Horseshoes				X	X	X	X	
• Scrollwork	X			X	X	X	X	

How Often Should You Train?

A common question is how often should the grip be trained. Your own body has the best answer. Each of us is a little different with our recovery time as well as gains in strength. As time progresses, you will learn your own best time clock.

When it comes to training your grip, I would suggest three times a week to start. Use a variety of exercises to get the best results. For instance, include an exercise to develop crushing strength, one for pinch gripping power, and one for holding strength. Once again, it is very important to learn your own body.

As a basis I would suggest doing five sets for crushing strength. For example, if you use a grip machine or a heavy-duty gripper, start with a couple of warm-up sets to get the circulation flowing into your lower arms. From there, use your last three sets for training with heavy weight or pressure.

As far as a pinch grip exercise, I would suggest using a weight that you can lift and hold for about five seconds. When you are able to hold the weight for ten seconds, it is time to add weight, if strength is your goal. Of course, for a goal of endurance, a longer period is required. Once in a while, I will hold a pinch grip for as long as I can. One day, with two Ivanko 25-lb. plates held on the smooth side, I was able to pinch grip and hold them for one minute, using only the index finger and thumb of my right hand.

The following tables will help you put together your training programs. Table A. tells you which type of grip strength is developed by each of the exercises in this book. For example, the grip machine trains your crushing grip; the lever lift works your wrist and forearm, and so on. Use this table to select different exercises that will help you develop all-around hand strength.

Table B. lays out some of the exercises that are especially suited to developing a superb grip for a sport or activity. You will want to emphasize these exercises in your training for that particular sport; for example, rock climbers will want to especially train their fingers and fingertips, arm wrestlers their wrists and forearms, and so on. Remember, though, that to develop a truly superior grip, you need to cross-train in all the areas of grip strength, so be sure to include exercises from all categories in your training.

Table C. gives you some sample workout routines. These are just guidelines. Feel free to modify them or make up your own depending

Table B.
Train on These Exercises in Particular
to Excel in These Athletic Areas

Martial Artist—fingers, fingertips, pinch grip
- Bag catching
- Fingertip push-ups
- Block weights, especially block toss
- Sand grabbing
- Baseball lift
- Titan's Telegraph Key

Arm Wrestler—crushing grip, wrist, forearm, overall lower arm
- Level lift or Weaver stick
- Rope climbing
- Wrist roller
- Wrist curls or weight plate curls
- Handgrippers or grip machine
- Thick-handled DB's
- Double hammer squeeze
- Block weights

Rodeo Rider—vise grip, wrist, forearm, overall lower arm
- One-hand muscle outs with bucket of sand
- Rope climbing
- Handgrippers or grip machine
- Wrist curls or weight plate curls
- Level lift or Weaver stick
- Double hammer squeeze

Rock Climber—fingers, fingertips, pinch grip, upper body
- Bag catching
- Finger walking
- Fingertip push-ups
- Titan's Telegraph Key
- Timber lifting or plate lifting
- Block weights
- Thick-handled DB's
- Rope climbing

Pianist, Harpist, Flutist—fingers, fingertips, pinch grip
- Finger walking
- Titan's Telegraph Key
- Individual finger lifts

Baseball Player—wrist, vise grip
- Lever lift or Weaver stick
- Baseball lift
- Wrist roller
- Handgrippers or grip machine

Bowler—wrist, fingers
- Wrist curls or weight plate curls
- Wrist roller
- Lever lift or Weaver stick
- Baseball lift

Table B. (continued)
Train on These Exercises in Particular
to Excel in These Athletic Areas

Football Player—pinch grip, vise grip, lower arm general
- Block weights
- Thick-handled DB's or kettlebells
- Handgrippers or grip machine
- Rope climbing
- Weight plate curls
- Baseball lift

Heavy Events Athlete—overall lower arm, vise grip
- Rope climbing
- Thick-handled DB's
- Kettlebells
- Handgrippers or grip machine
- Wrist curls or weight plate curls
- Baseball lift

Golfer—wrist, overall lower arm, upper body
- Lever lift or Weaver stick
- Thick-handled DB's
- Wrist curls or weight plate curls

Tennis Player—wrist, forearm, vise grip
- Lever lift or Weaver stick
- Wrist roller
- Baseball lift
- Wrist curls or weight plate curls
- Handgrippers or grip machine

Powerlifter—vise grip, overall lower arm, upper body
- Rope climbing
- Handgrippers or grip machine
- Thick-handled DB's
- Kettlebells

Olympic Weightlifter—vise grip, overall lower arm, upper body
- Rope climbing
- Thick-handled DB's
- Kettlebells
- Handgrippers or grip machine

Professional strongman—all grip areas
- Training program including all areas of grip, lower arm and upper body strength.

Archer—fingers, vise grip, wrists, upper body
- Titan's Telegraph Key
- Handgrippers or grip machine
- Finger walking
- Individual finger lifts
- Wrist roller
- Wrist curls or weight plate curls
- Rope climbing

upon your goals. You might even invent some exercises of your own or work in your old favorites.

Try to stick with a set of exercises for a while and improve your performance. Then move to another level or set of exercises and try to make progress with those. You might want to keep a training log with 1) your goals for that week, 2) the lifts and exercises in your workout,

---

Table C.
Sample Training Routines

Work on a routine for a few weeks, until you make some progress; then move on to another program at the same level or move up a level.

Beginner A:
• Warm-up
• Block weights: pick one or two exercises such as tossing, farmer's walk, clean and press, snatch lift, individual finger lifts, or follow the leader
• Heavy-duty handgrippers
• Wrist roller

Beginner B:
• Warm-up
• Grip machine
• Weight plate pinch gripping
• Wrist curls

Beginner C:
• Warm-up
• Titan's Telegraph Key
• Wire cutting
• Lever lift/Weaver stick

Intermediate A:
• Warm-up
• Block weights: pick two or three exercises such as tossing, farmer's walk, clean and press, snatch lift, individual finger lifts, or follow the leader
• Heavy-duty handgrippers
• Curling weight plates
• Rope climbing

Intermediate B:
• Warm-up
• Wide timber lifting: deadlifts, rows (upright or one-arm)
• Double hammer squeeze
• Pulling cut nails
• Baseball lift
• Kettlebells: swings, one-arm rows, tossing, etc.

Table C. (continued)
Sample Training Routines

Intermediate C:
- Warm-up
- Block weights: pick two or three exercises such as tossing, farmer's walk, clean and press, snatch lift, individual finger lifts, or follow the leader
- Mr. Pinch-O-Grip
- Plier lifting
- Lever lift/Weaver stick
- Thick-handled DB's: one-arm rows, curls, cleans, shrugs

Advanced A:
- Warm-up
- Block weights: pick four or five exercises such as tossing, farmer's walk, clean and press, snatch lift, individual finger lifts, or follow the leader
- Titan's Telegraph Key
- Anvil or axe head lifting
- Heavy-duty handgrippers
- Nail bending
- Wrist roller
- Baseball lift
- Thick-handled DB's: one-arm rows, curls, cleans, shrugs
- Finger extension—jar lifting

Advanced B:
- Warm-up
- Block weights: pick four or five exercises such as tossing, farmer's walk, clean and press, snatch lift, individual finger lifts, or follow the leader
- Grip machine
- Bag catching
- Fingertip push-ups
- Wrist curls
- Rope climbing
- Baseball lift
- Finger extension—sand bucket

Advanced C:
- Warm-up
- Wide timber lifting: deadlifts, rows (upright or one-arm)
- Mr. Pinch-O-Grip
- Wire cutting
- Sand grabbing
- Curling weight plates
- Rope climbing
- Kettlebells: swings, one-arm rows, tossing, etc.
- Finger extension bands

As you progress, start to work at some feats of strength like bar bending, scrollwork, bending nails, tearing cards, breaking horseshoes, coin bag carry, and the like.

and 3) a record of your actual workout. This will help you see where you are going, and you can adjust your goals each week as needed.

In my own training I do not do set routines or a certain amount of sets. I also do not watch the clock. I simply train the way I feel at the time. Once again, if you are truly serious about obtaining great grip strength, I suggest that you do a variety of exercises, hitting all the angles with an emphasis on the exercises that will help you with your sport or individual goal.

The main thing is to stay motivated. The best way for this is to set goals and consistently try to improve yourself working towards those goals, whether they are short or long-term.

Enjoy yourself, and good luck training.

Chapter Ten

The Vise Grip for Bending

For years now I've been bending steel, and I'm always asked what does it take to bend steel. Well, first of all, there are many types of steel-bending. Of course there are nails that can be bent. People seem to be the most interested in bending nails. However, there are many other objects such as steel bars and horseshoes, as well as the art of iron coiling or scrollwork. This scrollwork, as we will call it, is the bending of steel bars into artistic designs. It is a great workout for the lower arms, as well as a great demonstration of strength.

Any type of real steel bending calls for a very tight grip or, you may say, a vise grip. For instance, if you put a piece of steel into a good heavy-duty shop vise and tighten the vise tightly on the steel, you will find that the piece of steel becomes much easier to bend. You may say, "Oh, everyone knows that." However, many people forget this principle when they think about bending steel in their hands.

Many of the world's strongest men are unable to bend even the least tempered nail. Often I run across huge powerful men in programs where I am performing feats of strength. They come up to me after the show and want to try and bend something, usually a nail. They huff and puff on a hard nail and they can't believe that they can't even put a dent or kink in the nail. About this time, they usually tell me how much they can bench press or how much they curled last week.

After this, they want to know if I have a softer nail. At times I carry a regular or softer nail—this is a nail that is generally your typical hardware nail that is not hardened or tempered. They take a good look at this nail, grasp it, and again they blow into it with everything they have, with the same outcome—they can't do anything with it. They usually walk off in a state of disbelief that they couldn't bend the nails— after all, they had won powerlifting meets.

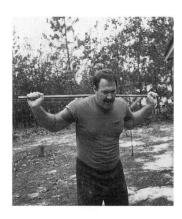

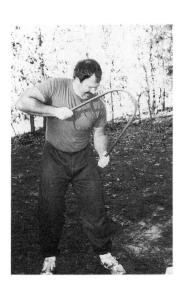

John bends a 3/4 inch steel bar. Photos by Steve Jeck.

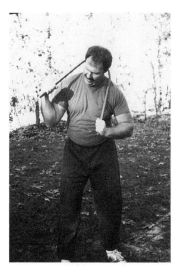

The fact that these men failed is not that they aren't strong. They are very strong. However, there are many types of strength and the strength for bending steel is somewhat different than the strength for lifting heavy barbells. The fact is that there are only a handful of good steel benders in the world today. It is a lost art. Many of the old strongmen on stage were good steel benders, mainly because of their lower arm strength.

Back to the vise illustration: When a piece of steel is placed into a tight vise, it is completely secured. There is no slip or slide in the vise's grasp. Once in this secure state, you can use your strength to bend the steel. If the vise is not tightened securely, the steel will move or slip when you attempt to bend it. This is the same principle when you are bending a nail. There is a certain amount of slip in the grip being applied to the nail. The strongest hands in the world are not completely secure like the vise. However, the tighter the grip, the more actual strength can be applied. The strongest upper body in the world cannot get leverage on a nail if the grip is not secure.

I will give you a crazy example. An old strongman once told me that he was stronger than a tree in the woods. We were standing at the edge of the forest so I, of course, said, "Which tree?"

He replied, "The largest tree in the forest." Before I could say anything else, he said that he could prove it.

"How?" I asked.

"I can bend a nail or a horseshoe and the tree can't. This of course makes me the stronger."

He certainly had a point. This unusual comparison made me aware of just how important the hands are, and without the grasp of the hands, not a whole lot can be accomplished. Somehow most of the modern day athletes have gotten caught up in how big their chest is or what their biceps measure. They have forgotten they have hands, so to speak.

Another interesting point to be made is that as powerful and awesome as a hurricane is, it does not have the strength to bend a nail or horseshoe either. Please forgive my two strange comparisons, but it is the truth and it must be completely understood if you ever expect to be a great bender of steel.

Now that my point has been made, let's look at three types of bending, all of which are related, but yet very different. We will start with nail bending. Out of all the letters and calls I get, nail bending seems to be one of the most popular conversations. People either want to know how to train to bend nails or they want some bent nails for a conversation piece. First of all, most strongmen bend the classic 60-penny nail, which is a six-inch nail 1/4 inch thick. Only the strongest of the strong bend bigger nails like 80- or 100-penny nails.

If you wish to work on nail bending, I would suggest you purchase 40-penny nails to start. They are easier to bend and they will help you get a feel for what you're trying to accomplish. For safety's sake you may want to cut off the point of the nail with a hacksaw or, to make it easier, cut it off with bolt cutters. It is best to cover the nail with an old washcloth or shop rag. Use enough cloth to protect your hands, but do not use so much covering that you cannot get a secure grip. This will be defeating the purpose, and I will be back to telling you more stories about trees and hurricanes.

This is a book about the development of the lower arms, not a book on how to bend nails, so I won't try to teach you how to bend them, for this would be very lengthy. I have, however, told you about the material it takes to get started. It will probably feel awkward at first, but with practice you will get a feel for it. Nail bending is a great way to develop strong tendons and ligaments in the wrist and forearms.

I will show you a good exercise for developing hand strength for nail bending. If you think about the thickness of a nail, even a thick spike, you will realize that the nail is much thinner than any bar you will ever grip, especially a thick-handled dumbbell or block weight. In normal circumstances, it would be rare that you ever grip anything as thin as a nail with your whole hand.

To start your new exercise you will need a thin piece of rope. You can go to the hardware and purchase several feet of rope that is about 1/4 inch thick; or, in other words, a rope that is about as thick as your nail. If you have to, you can use a piece of baling twine, or basically anything that is thin and close to your nail in size.

Tie your rope around a smaller dumbbell or, if you don't have dumbbells, use a five-gallon bucket of sand or water. After you have tied one end of the rope around the handle, let the other end of the rope remain straight and untied. You will now reach out and grasp the rope with one hand, as if you're reaching out to grab onto a pole. The rope should be vertical or straight up and down throughout the entire move-ment, and your arm straight out in front of you. Now lift the dumbbell or bucket off the ground by simply lifting up on the rope. This is like performing a muscle out. Hold the weight as long as you can in this position. This is a rare way to train your grip, one you probably haven't done or even seen before. It will work your hand in a way that is very similar to nail bending. It will help you to tightly grip objects the size of nails.

If you are serious about nail bending, I would strongly suggest that you use this exercise in your routine. Gradually add weight to this exercise, and also work at holding the weight out by the rope for as long as possible. As with all exercises, train each hand equally.

Another type of bending that is a show stopper is the bending of steel bars into designs, called scrollwork. Scrollwork is rarely seen any more. I often bend scrolls in my programs and it is always a way to capture the audience. I have done many designs—sometimes I bend the bar into a

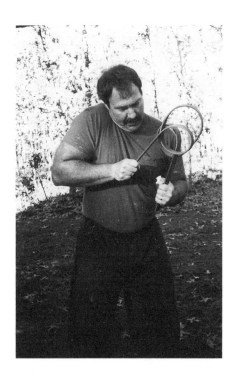

John demonstrates the traditional strongman art of scrollwork. Photo by Steve Jeck.

three-leaf clover or maybe the letter M from the alphabet, or sometimes I just scroll the bar into a coil of circles.

Scrolling steel develops powerful fingers and wrists. Much endurance is needed to finish a scroll without stopping to rest. For practicing bar scrolling, I like to use a piece of 1/2-inch round hot rolled steel. Scrolling the bar very tightly is when a really viselike grip comes into play.

The famous Polish strongman Siegmund Breitbart used to challenge blacksmiths, betting them that he could bend a very strong piece of steel into a design with his hands quicker than they could make the design with their hammers, tongs, and anvil. Breitbart always won. Breitbart was one of the best steel benders of all time.

The last type of bending we will discuss is the bending and breaking of horseshoes. This bend, I feel, is the most difficult for it requires overall strength in the entire arms and shoulders. I mentioned earlier in the chapter about old-time strongmen who bent and broke horseshoes. This feat is truly an amazing feat in its true sense—I say true sense because all horseshoes are not tempered, and you may be able to find a shoe that bends very easily.

When I am asked about the strength of horseshoes, I often find it hard to explain, for they can vary from shoe to shoe. Some shoes that are large are not always as strong as thinner ones. It all depends on the steel, not the size. I always bend used horseshoes, because new ones are very expensive. They usually cost between seven and ten dollars a shoe. As you can see, this would be an expensive habit to get into. However, there is a racetrack close to my house that shoes many horses all year long. When they change the horseshoes, they throw the old shoes out back behind the building. With horseshoes you will find that the type of steel used does not lose its strength for a long time. So even though when I pick up these horseshoes out of a pile, they may be a little rusty, their strength is the same as when they were new. If you wish to scrub them a little with steel wool, all the rust will come off.

You may be able to find a place that boards horses in your area. If not, look for someone who owns horses; they will probably let you have the old horseshoes. One more tip—you can also find a farrier or black-smith by looking in your local Yellow Pages.

Once you find some horseshoes, be sure to remove any nail tacks for they will ruin your day if they poke into your hand. Also, be sure to use washcloths or old rags to bend the horseshoes. Once again as with the nails, I will not try to teach you how to bend horseshoes—it would be too lengthy. Remember, an extremely strong grip and powerful fore-arms are required to bend a forged horseshoe. It will be good training for you even if the horseshoe does not budge, so hang in there.

I have briefly explained three types of steel bending. All are great training for the lower arms; however, all of the three require different movements, working the grip in a different way. You will find that to master these types of bends, you will need to develop a viselike grip.

Chapter Eleven

Testing Your Endurance: Can You Muster This?

I am often asked about different feats of hand and wrist strength. A popular question is what feats of strength do I feel are the most difficult. This question of course is nearly impossible to answer. However, many feats of strength come to mind. In this chapter I have picked out five feats of strength that involve the hand and wrist. These feats also involve objects that are easy to find without much expense. It is safe to say that if you can accomplish each of these feats, you have truly amazing lower arm strength. If you are able to do even one or two of them, you have accomplished a lot. Our question here is, "Can you muster this?"

Our first feat involves an ordinary potato, a raw potato. As a matter of fact a raw potato is all you'll need for this first feat. Now all you have to do is squeeze the potato into a pulp with one hand. That's it. Doesn't sound that hard, does it? Simply grasp it with one hand and attempt to crush it as you would a handgripper or a rubber ball.

If you have ever tried to close the IronMind #3 gripper—you know, the one that takes almost 300 lbs. of pressure to close—if you have tried, I will just tell you I think the potato is harder to crush than the gripper. Also, the potato will remain hard even as your fingers start to penetrate the surface. I have crushed a potato a handful of times, with a tremendous battle.

If your fingernails are at all long, be sure to trim them, for the potato is so hard it may break them off if you try to dig in with your fingers. This feat used to be performed by Robert Vickers of England. When people first think of crushing a potato in their hand they think it sounds easy, but they are usually thinking of a baked potato instead of a raw potato. This feat will call on every ounce of your gripping power. If you don't succeed you can always bake the potato.

The next feat of grip strength will test your endurance as well as your strength. In Chapter 8. on manual labor, I mentioned the icemen who delivered the heavy blocks of ice by carrying them with a set of ice tongs. I also mentioned August Johnson, an iceman who once carried a 32-lb. bag of coins in one hand for a full mile. He did not hold the bag against his body or shift the bag from hand to hand. He just kept the same grip on the bag for the entire mile.

This feat is your next challenge. It may not sound that hard to carry 32 lbs. for a mile; however, it is truly an amazing accomplishment. When you try this one—and I have a feeling you will try it—if you can't find a bag large enough to hold 32 lbs., you can use a five-gallon bucket or even a garden bucket to carry. Load it up with 32 lbs. of dirt or sand. Now you will have to take a towel or a large cloth and tie it around the handle of the bucket. Grasp the towel with one hand, as though you were going to wring water out of it. You will keep this grip on the towel and carry the 32-lb. bucket for one mile without changing hands or setting the bucket down. This is the manner in which August Johnson gripped the bag of coins. No handle, just by gripping the cloth. It will probably not take long for your hand to fatigue in this type of grip. This is truly a tremendous feat of hand strength.

The third challenge feat is a little different from the first two feats, in which you were able to use your whole hand. This feat requires tremendous finger strength as well as thumb strength. You will need a pack of plastic-coated poker cards. Anywhere you go you will probably find the plastic-coated cards. The paper cards which the old-timers used are nearly impossible to find anymore.

Take the full deck of cards and attempt to tear the corner off the deck. Try to tear a chunk about the size of a quarter off the corner of the deck. I have been performing this for years now and it always seems to amaze any audience. The old vaudeville strongman Harold Ansorge used to perform this feat. His feat is still displayed in the famous Ripley's *Believe It or Not* book.

As you try to duplicate this feat, you will notice that you are only able to get a grip on the cards with your thumb and the tips of your index and forefingers. After you get a grasp on the corner of the cards, try to start a small tear in the corner. If you get a tear started, then try to pull off the corner of the cards. If you do not like the feel of pulling off the corner, you can try to twist off the corner. This is a little different technique that you can try. Either way, you will have to have fingertip strength as well as endurance to be successful with this feat, for it is extremely difficult.

Just for fun, try to tear off the corner of the cards with a pair of pliers; this will show you how difficult the feat really is. Grasp the cards with your left hand to secure the cards and use the pliers to grip the corner. Now try to pull or twist the corner off with the pliers.

When you can master the feat of tearing off the corners of a deck of poker cards, you can be sure that you have a grip of steel.

Another feat that deserves special mention is a feat that is very rare and involves curling weight plates (see Chapter 7.) It is a feat that requires great finger strength as well as great wrist strength. Looking back in the old books about strongmen, you would occasionally find where a strongman could lift a 50-lb. weight plate in one hand using a pinch grip and then curl the weight to his chest. This curl is, of course, done with the palm of the hand facing upward and the weight lying over the top of the hand. This puts the weight in a position that tasks your wrist and hand to the utmost. This feat of strength is world class in any book. The average man cannot curl a 25-lb. weight plate in this manner, and it takes a very strong-handed man to curl a 35-lb. plate. So just imagine a 50-lb. plate and the pressure on the wrist that goes with it. Also, it's not only the weight of the plate that makes it harder, but also as the weight gets heavier the plate gets longer, making the leverage work against you.

When you try this one, be sure to warm up your wrist first, and also be sure to try a smaller weight plate first, like a 25-lb. plate. Special note: This exercise is a great way to build the wrist and fingers; however, it is also a way to strain your wrist if it is overdone. So, once again, warm up and start slowly. To mention a special performance of this feat, Clevio Massimo could curl a 50-lb. weight plate with either hand for ten repetitions. This exercise or feat of strength, depending on the amount of weight that is used, may be one of the greatest ways to develop the tendons and ligaments in the wrist and the hand, so start curling those weight plates.

The fifth feat of lower arm strength requires amazing forearm and wrist strength. This feat is also a feat that I've been doing in demonstrations for many years now. Most of the time people can hardly believe that I can accomplish this feat.

You will need a washcloth or shop rag for this one. You will also need an ordinary 60-penny nail. This nail can be purchased at most hardware stores, and is six inches in length and 1/4-inch thick in diameter. Wrap the nail in the cloth and place it behind your back. Next, grasp the nail with both hands and attempt to bend it downward with your hands.

As you will surely find out, this is no easy feat. There is no leverage whatsoever and your wrists and hands are all you have to use. You can find no angle to gain shoulder or arm strength. All the strength must be in the wrists.

People often ask me if you need to be flexible to do this feat. You don't need to be overly flexible; however, if you are very tight in your shoulders and chest you may have trouble in this position. If you feel tight or cramped in this position, you may want to lean back a little by simply arching your back. This will give you a little more freedom to attempt to bend the nail.

This feat is very difficult. I have never heard of anyone ever doing this feat with a 60-penny nail, other than myself. If you practice it for a while, you will become more comfortable in this position. You can also try to tear poker cards and telephone books with your hands behind your back. All of these objects are hard to handle with your hands behind your back, but I feel bending the 60-penny nail is the most difficult.

Well, these are the five feats of hand and wrist strength I have chosen. There are of course many others that could be mentioned as well. I picked these five for their difficulty, but I also chose them because they involve objects easy to obtain, and they also do not involve much expense. If you are able to accomplish any or all of these feats of strength, drop me a line and tell me about it. Who knows, next time I might be writing about you.

Chapter Twelve

Are These For Real? — You Be the Judge

As a professional strongman, I have been involved in the strength world for a long time now. I've been performing feats of strength for about eighteen years. You could say I've seen it all. There are a handful of questions that seem to crop up quite regularly pertaining to certain feats of strength.

In this chapter, we will look at four feats of strength that seem to be talked about often, but are never seen in real life. Are they for real or are they simply fairy tales? We will take a good look at them and what it takes to accomplish such feats.

First let's look at the feat of coin bending or breaking. What an enigma. Everywhere I go to perform, someone comes up to me after the show and starts talking about someone who either bends or breaks coins with his fingers. Often they tell me that the person bends or breaks the coins by holding the coin with one hand and crushing it with his index finger and thumb like a bottle cap. I always ask the person telling the story where the coin bender is from and just who he is. This is where the fun usually begins. The person has either moved away or the person was just someone they met in passing. No matter who tells the story, he can never tell you where you can find this master of finger strength. One gets the feeling that you are searching for the Abominable Snowman or perhaps searching for a pot of gold at the end of the rainbow.

In all seriousness, there were a number of strongmen who used to bend or break coins. These strongmen were from the old days, and the coins were not as strong then. Also, these strongmen were not from America. The coins of Britain, France, and other countries were not as strong as our American coins of today.

I have gone to many coin shops and purchased many coins from other countries and found for the most part that our coins are much harder in substance than the coins from other countries—the English penny for instance. You know, the one that Charles Vansittart (known as "The Man with the Iron Grip") used to bend. These coins are not the size of our penny. They are slightly larger than our 50-cent piece or more like our silver dollars of old. William Caswell was a small man, but a master of finger strength. Caswell could bend and break these coins in many different manners.

I speak of Vansittart and Caswell with all respect for they were men of great grip strength. However, before you see these feats as impossible you must again realize that these coins were much larger than people of today realize and that the metal of these coins was not as strong as today's coins. Yes, I truly believe a strong-fingered man could bend and also break English pennies and also some other European coins. As for our American coins of today, it is questionable.

I think I'll let you decide how hard it would be to bend a quarter double, or how hard it would be to break the same quarter. Find a quarter that you can spare. Even a borrowed quarter will do. Find two pairs of pliers and grip one half of the quarter with one pair of the pliers and grip the other half of the quarter with the other pair. Now by grasping the handles of the pliers, start bending the quarter back and forth. See how many times back and forth it takes to break the quarter. Notice how much leverage you have with both pairs of pliers. Also, notice how secure the grip is with both pairs of pliers. Now think how many times it takes, you going back and forth, until the quarter breaks.

As I said earlier, the choice is yours whether you think it is possible to break an American coin with just the fingers or not. Like myself, I'm sure you have heard stories of people able to do such a feat. So, next time someone comes up to you and tells you of a past experience he had seeing a person breaking coins with his fingers, you can either politely smile and nod, or you can ask them if they believe in vampires too.

The second feat of grip strength that we will examine is the feat of squeezing a tennis ball until it bursts or explodes. This is not the same as tearing a tennis ball in two. Tearing a tennis ball in half is very difficult, but not impossible. Grasping the ball and trying to start a tear in the seam is how you would accomplish this feat. It is easily one of the hardest feats of hand strength that can be tackled.

I mention this feat of tearing the tennis ball in half because it is often confused with the feat of squeezing the ball until it explodes. I discussed above Charles Vansittart in the coin-breaking section. Vansittart was said also to be able to squeeze a tennis ball until it exploded.

Once again, I can tell you that tennis balls in the early 1900s were made differently than the tennis balls of today. I have asked several tennis professionals if they knew the exact makeup of the original tennis balls. None of the tennis pros knew for sure, but they all said that the balls were not nearly as durable back then. I truly believe that Vansittart could do this feat with the earlier tennis balls.

In the last several years I have come across five or six different people, all from different areas, that say they have seen someone squeeze a tennis ball until it exploded—a new tennis ball, as well. I have clamped onto a tennis ball, squeezing with all my might for as long as I could on several occasions, only to find the tennis ball springing back to life looking as good as new.

To research this feat some more, I decided to take a brand-new tennis ball and place it into a shop vise. I tightened the vise so that the ball was completely collapsed and that the ends of the vise were touching, so that the tennis ball was completely crushed under the pressure of the vise. I placed the tennis ball in the vise on a Friday afternoon. I went away for the weekend and returned on Monday morning. I loosened the vise and the ball that had been completely crushed in the vise for the entire weekend sprang back to life once again. I tried this same experiment with another brand of tennis ball. Again the same results. Once again, I will let you be the judge of this feat and whether or not it can be accomplished.

The third feat of grip strength that is often brought up is the squeezing of a metal can until the top bursts off. This has always been a feat that has been talked about from construction sites to barrooms. This is also a feat that I have never seen done in real life. As you know, it is always easily done on TV, but in real life the performers of this feat are as elusive as the coin breakers.

There are many different types of cans on the market and some are made of tougher metal than others. Most cans of today seem to be a little thinner than the metal cans of the past; however, the soda cans of today are still very durable. Many people squeeze the cans after they are empty, and of course the cans easily collapse. They think if they can crush the can so easily with it being empty, they can surely squeeze a full can with the top still secured, until the top bursts with the pressure. This may not be so easily done.

About a year ago, I decided to conduct a test on a full can of Coke similar to the test I conducted on the tennis balls. I placed a full can of Coke on its side on the ground in my driveway. From there I drove a pickup truck on top of the can. I placed the tire on the can, so that the weight of the vehicle was directly on the middle of the can. This would be in a similar position to that of the hand applying pressure to the middle of the can when squeezing it.

Of course the can completely collapsed under the great pressure of the pickup truck. However, the top of the can remained intact. I conducted this test with several different soda cans. A couple of times the can was crushed so flat that a small crease was started in the middle of the can. This allowed the liquid to leak out under the great pressure. Also the top of the can bowed out and even stretched under the pressure, but every time the top remained intact, with no leak in the top of the can.

There may be some cans on the market with a cheaper or less durable metal. I didn't find any myself. Once again, we have a feat of hand strength that remains a mystery.

The fourth and final feat of strength we will examine is a feat of total upper body strength with an emphasis on the lower arms. Is there anybody out there involved in the strength field who hasn't been told by someone, that they knew of or heard of someone who could bend railroad spikes with his hands?

You know, the real railroad spikes—not the 100-penny nails or the 80-penny nails, but the real railroad spikes. The real railroad spikes are a little less than six inches long, square in shape, and 5/8 inches in diameter, with a very large head. These spikes are exclusively used on the railroad. I have been told that a long time ago some railroad spikes were much longer. I have never seen the longer ones myself. However, if these spikes of years ago were around ten inches long, it would be possible to bend them. This would still be extremely difficult. In my years of bending steel and also researching the steel benders of the past and present, it is my opinion that only about ten men of past or present would even have a chance of bending these spikes if they were ten inches long.

The 100-penny nails of present times are ten inches long and 3/8-inch in diameter. They are round in shape. Only a few hardware stores carry them anymore. I have been bending them in acts for a number of years now. Most 100-penny nails are made of pretty good steel and are very hard to bend.

Other than myself, the only other man I know of that can bend 100-penny nails is Slim "The Hammerman" Farman. Slim is the greatest sledgehammer lifter of all time and also, easily one of the greatest strongmen of all time. There are two or three other men whom I have heard of that are said to be able to bend these nails; however, I have never personally witnessed their doing so.

My point here is that the 100-penny nails that are ten inches long and 3/8-inch diameter are extremely hard to bend. So just imagine the traditional railroad spike that is only slightly over half the length of the 100-penny nail. Also, remember the railroad spike is much thicker than the 100-penny nail. I have met a couple of men who said they could bend a railroad spike. Both of these men tried to bend a 60-penny nail that was made of moderately tough steel. Both of these fellows were unable to put even a bow in these nails. I would have to estimate that a railroad spike would be about four times as hard to bend as these 60-penny nails.

Once again you tell me if this feat of strength is possible or not. If anyone truly knows of anyone who can perform any of these four feats of strength, please let me know and I'll certainly put them in my next book. Until then these feats will be in the same category as the lepre-chauns of Ireland and the werewolves of London.

How to Make Your Own Thick-Handled Dumbbells

You may have always wondered how you could purchase an old-time thick-handled dumbbell. Well, the truth is you probably can't.* You may find a craftsman at a machine shop that you could talk into giving it a try, or maybe if you are wealthy you could possibly find an old-time collector who has one for a great price. However, if you are not rich or you don't want to spend months and hundreds of dollars purchasing one, I will show you how you can make your own.

Whether you work out at a gym or home, you have probably noticed that there are several dumbbells on the market that are simply a cast weight, one that doesn't require collars and cannot be changed to increase or lessen the weight. These dumbbells are usually just the block type weights with a bar or handle in the middle. All that is needed is to find this type of dumbbell to make your new tool of grip success. Many large sporting goods stores will carry these types of dumbbells.

The York Barbell Company puts out heavy cast dumbbells of this sort as well as the Ivanko Company. You will also find many cast hexhead dumbbells on the market. Any of these weights will work. Personally, I like to use the York dumbbells for the task, but any of these others will work.

Now many of you are wondering how are we going to make these thin normal-sized handles into thick-handled ones—perhaps a magic trick. No, something much easier. Simply pick out a dumbbell you like and from here all you need to do is cut off the handle, leaving you with the two block weights. You can have a welder burn off the handle or a machinist will probably have a special saw that will do the job. My favorite way is to take a hacksaw and cut off the bar. This is also a good

Editor's Note: If you can forego the old-time look of a one-piece dumbbell, you might appreciate the practical advantages of a plate-loading thick-handled dumbbell, which you can make or buy.

hand workout. If you choose this method it will probably take you about forty minutes to cut off both ends. Try to cut off the ends right neat to the ball. Using the hacksaw is of course the cheapest way to go, but the others won't cost much either.

Now that you are looking at two blocks of iron, the next step is to find a thick handle. If you go to a welding shop or to a steel company or even to a large machine shop, you will be able to find round thick steel or iron pipes. Pick out a piece of pipe. Now this piece of pipe needs to be welded to the two block weights from your dumbbell, and this, of course, gives you a new handle. This handle will have to be welded by a professional welder.* He will be able to weld this on very quickly and easily, which makes the expense to you reasonable. You may also want the welder to cut off the original handle from your weight so you won't have to use a hacksaw. He can probably cut off the handle and weld your new piece of pipe on in a few short minutes, here again making your expense low.

The big question of course is how thick a piece of pipe needs to be welded on and how heavy does your dumbbell need to be. You don't want something that is too light to help you or something so heavy and awkward you can't even lift it off the floor.

First, let's address the problem of the thickness. You will not want a handle less than two inches in diameter, as this would be defeating the purpose. You will also not want a handle over three inches in diameter unless you have a gigantic hand—not a big hand, but gigantic. If you use a shaft that is way too big, it can put excessive stress on the thumb. So we are shooting for something from two inches to three inches in diameter. An important note to remember is that most of the famous strongmen of the past used dumbbells with a handle around 2-1/2 inches thick. This is also my advice to you. If you have small hands, a two-inch shaft may be best; if you have exceptionally large hands, a three-inch shaft will be all right. For a person with normal-sized hands, let's stick to 2-1/2 inches.

When you go to buy your pipe you will probably be able to find a pipe that is 2-1/2 inches thick; most larger steel companies or machine shops will have pipe that jumps every 1/4 or 1/2 inch. If you make several calls and can't find pipe that ranges every 1/4 to 1/2 inch and you

*Editor's Note: Welding steel to iron really isn't desirable; it should never be used where life or limb depends on the weld holding.

are in a hurry to get started, you can get a two-inch diameter pipe and use tape around the shaft to thicken it. Adhesive tape is best, but duct tape will also work.

Our next question is how heavy a dumbbell should be used. For training you will have to remember that a dumbbell with a thick handle feels much heavier than a dumbbell with a normal handle. I would say that a man with a good grip would probably want to train with a dumb-bell of about 50 to 70 lbs. on a 2-1/2 inch handle. This training would consist of exercises like one-arm rows, shrugs, curls, and cleans. A very strong man with a great grip could probably train with more. If you haven't used weights much or you don't have very strong hands, I would start with a weight of around 30 lbs.

How to Make Your Own Kettlebells

Now to make our kettlebells we will look at two methods. First the more expensive way. Once again we will be using block weights. Pick out the size you want; for instance, if you want two 30-lb. kettlebells you will need a 60-lb. dumbbell, or if you wish to have two 50-lb. kettlebells you will need a 100-lb. dumbbell. As with the thick-handled dumbbells you will need to pick out a dumbbell that is a block weight fashion, and not a plate or disc style dumbbell. The York dumbbells are by far the best for our project, but the Ivanko or the hexagon weights will also work.

Once again you will have to cut off the ends of your weight with either a hacksaw or the help of a welder or machinist. Now you have to pick out two pieces of steel to weld to the sides of your block weight. These pieces of steel will extend from the sides of the weight to the handle. It is best to use a flat piece of steel about 3/4-inch by 1/4-inch, but if this is hard for you to find, you may also use a round piece of steel for the job. Even retaining wall steel 1/2-inch thick will work. The length of steel that is to be welded from the sides of the weight to the sides of the handle will vary with the size of the kettlebell. You will have to decide how long a handle you want.

For your handle I would suggest a round steel pipe of about two to 2-1/2 inches in diameter. This again can be purchased at a machine shop, steel company, or even at a welder's shop. You will need two short pieces of pipe for your handles, assuming you want a pair of kettlebells instead of just one. Once again, your two pieces of steel will be welded to the sides of the block weight, and then the other end of the pieces of steel will be welded to the ends of your handle. If there are any questions how to make this type of kettlebell, please look closely at the kettlebell in the photo (next page) to clearly understand. It is a 56-lb. kettlebell with a handle three inches thick.

The other way of making kettlebells is much cheaper but will work just as well. This method of craftsmanship will not win any awards at an art gallery. However, if it's results you want and you don't want to spend a lot of money, this may be the way for you.

First of all, you will need to find a five-gallon bucket. The bucket must be plastic, not metal. You can probably find an old five-gallon bucket on a construction site that they may let you have, or you can go to a hardware store or a lumber yard and purchase one. Next, while you are at the hardware store or lumber yard, you will need to purchase some

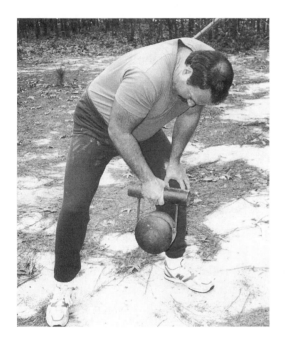

John does some one-arm bentover rows with his homemade 56-lb. kettlebell; the handle is three inches thick. Photo by Steve Jeck.

ready-mixed concrete. This concrete comes in bags of 50 pounds. This is the type of concrete that is already mixed with sand, and you simply need to add water and stir a little. It will usually take a full day to completely harden. The amount of concrete you will need depends on the weight of your kettlebells and also on how many kettlebells you want to make. A 50-lb. bag of ready-mixed concrete is of course going to weigh 50 pounds when poured out of the bag. When it is mixed with water it will weigh slightly more. If you are going to make two kettlebells, you will also need two five-gallon buckets. If you want three kettlebells you will need three buckets, and so on.

You have probably already figured out that you are going to pour and mix the concrete in your bucket. To give you a good idea of the weight that the five-gallon bucket will hold, I can remember my days working for the state highway, mixing concrete by hand. I used to like to carry the buckets completely full of concrete. One day we weighed the buckets completely full of concrete. We were surprised to find out that a five-gallon bucket full of concrete weighs about 80 to 85 pounds. This will be a good gauge for you to go by. So if you want a large kettlebell of around 85 pounds not counting the handle, fill your bucket to the top. Half of a bucket will weigh around 40 pounds, not counting the handle. A lot of you will want a kettlebell around 50 or 60 pounds. This will make it easy, because our 50-lb. bag of concrete plus water and handle will be around 60 pounds.

You will now need to go to the metal shop to get a handle. You can get a thick pipe again to have a thick-handled kettlebell. Get a short piece of pipe plus two pieces of steel that need to be welded to the pipe, as described above for the block weight kettlebell. They need to be welded just like the handle in the photo of the block weight kettlebell.

When you have all the materials needed, the hard part has been completed. Remember, your bucket or buckets must be plastic not metal. You're now ready to start. The first step is to put a long narrow slit in the bucket so that the bucket can later be cut off without difficulty. You can drill a small hole or two in the plastic. Now you use a razor knife or even a regular knife to make a couple of small narrow slits in the side of the bucket.

Pour your ready-mixed concrete into the bucket and add some water. Take a stick or shovel and stir the two together until they are mixed together. Try to level the top fairly evenly, although it will probably level out pretty evenly on its own. As you will see, the mix is pretty loose at first, but as it starts to harden you will need to place the prongs of the handle into the concrete. This will probably be several hours before you are ready to place the handle into the bucket—you will have to judge this for yourself. The concrete will need to be setting up pretty well before you set the handle. If the handle starts to sink into the mix, it is too loose and needs to set some more.

Once you get the handle set where you want, you will need to let the concrete set up completely. This will take about 24 hours. When the concrete is set you are ready to remove the bucket from the set concrete. Use a chisel or a large nail to pry the plastic loose. This is why you made the slits in the plastic. If the plastic is stubborn and doesn't want to come loose, you may need to use a pair of tin snips or wire cutters to start a good cut where you made your original slits.

Once you have removed the bucket you will notice you have a primitive, but very effective kettlebell complete with handle. You may want to sand the concrete to make it smoother. Special note: Be sure to set the prongs of the handle far enough down in the concrete to secure a strong bond. I would suggest a good four inches, especially with a heavy kettlebell.

John Brookfield enjoys performing and excels at a variety of traditional feats of strength. One of his recent performances was recognized by the *Guiness Book of World Records*.

The object of the record was to take seven different objects and bend, break or tear them as quickly as possible. The seven different feats were as follows:

1) Break ten cinder blocks with his elbow. The blocks were stacked on top of one another.

2) Tear a deck of plastic-coated poker cards wrapped in four layers of duct tape.

3) Bend double a large eight-inch file guaranteed for a lifetime.

4) Bend double a carriage bolt 3/8 inch in diameter and seven inches long. This bolt required a little over 500 lbs. of pressure to bend.

5) Break a pair of pliers; the pliers had a bolt placed between the jaws, which spread the handles, allowing the pliers to be squeezed like a handgripper. The handles snapped under the grip pressure.

6) Bend double two 40-penny nails wrapped together in duct tape.

7) Bend a steel bar 19 inches long and 1/2 inch thick. The bar was bent around his neck.

All of these objects were bent, torn, or broken in exactly 25.6 seconds total.